Fast Facts

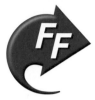

Fast Facts:
Obesity

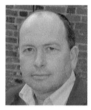

David Haslam MB BS DGM
Chair, National Obesity Forum
Senior Partner, Watton Place Clinic
Watton-at-Stone, Hertfordshire, UK
Physician in Obesity Medicine
Luton & Dunstable Hospital, Luton, UK

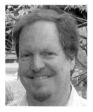

Gary Wittert MBBch MD FRACP
Mortlock Professor of Medicine
Head, School of Medicine
University of Adelaide
Senior Consultant Endocrinologist
Royal Adelaide Hospital
South Australia, Australia

Declaration of Independence
This book is as balanced and as practical as we can make it.
Ideas for improvement are always welcome: feedback@fastfacts.com

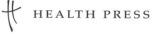 HEALTH PRESS

Fast Facts: Obesity
First published September 2009

FSC
Mixed Sources
Product group from well-managed
forests and other controlled sources

Cert no. SGS-COC-005493
www.fsc.org
© 1996 Forest Stewardship Council

Introduction

Obesity, particularly severe obesity, is highly prevalent in both adults and children.

As well as being a disease in its own right, obesity is a key risk factor for serious chronic conditions – notably type 2 diabetes mellitus, cardiovascular disease and many cancers – and also leads to a plethora of non-fatal but debilitating health problems, including musculoskeletal problems (e.g. osteoarthritis), respiratory problems, obstructive sleep apnea, and lower urinary tract and reproductive problems.

This new *Fast Facts* title has been written for people working at the coal face of primary care, who can play a key role in both preventing and treating obesity. It will also be useful to medical students and junior doctors who want to understand the causes and consequences of obesity. It describes the management of obesity, the three cornerstones of which are diet, physical activity and behavioral management, and also details the pharmacological and surgical approaches. Behavioral management, although something of a mystery to many clinicians, is critical to the success of obesity management, as it provides the key to changing patients' habits and attitudes to food and physical activity, and their ability to deal with stress, which are important for health and wellbeing irrespective of weight change.

Epidemiology

A global problem

The average body mass index (BMI) has been rising steadily since around 1900 as public health and nutrition have improved, but an even more rapid response in the last three decades has led to staggering rates of obesity worldwide, such that globally in 2005:

- approximately 1.6 billion adults (aged 15 years and over) were overweight (BMI > 25 kg/m^2)
- at least 400 million adults were obese (> 30 kg/m^2)
- at least 20 million children under 5 years of age were overweight.

The latest data from the US National Center for Health Statistics show that 30% of US adults (20 years of age and older) are obese – over 60 million people.

Although levels of obesity vary in different populations and are generally higher in developed countries (Figure 1.1), no region in the world is free from obesity and its related problems. Rates range from less than 5% in China, Japan and certain African nations to over 75% in urban Samoa. However, even in countries with a relatively low prevalence such as China, rates are still as high as 20% in some cities.

It is becoming clear that waist (abdominal) circumference is a more accurate predictor than BMI of an individual's risk of obesity-related cardiovascular and metabolic complications (see Chapter 2). Table 1.1 gives the prevalence of obesity measured by waist circumference in various countries and shows that the true prevalence of high-risk obesity is being significantly underestimated by reliance on BMI.

A growing problem

The prevalence of obesity in England (as measured by BMI) was about 24% in both men and women in 2007, and is expected to rise to 26% and 28%, respectively, by 2010. Figure 1.2 shows the striking increase in obesity across the USA between 1990 and 2007. Parallel increases are being seen in England, demonstrating the fate in store for the UK over the next decade or so unless the management of obesity improves.

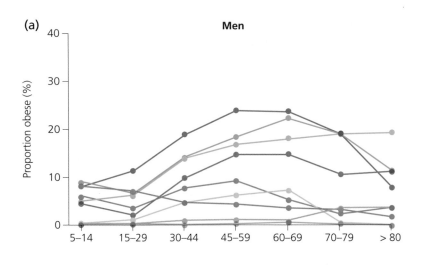

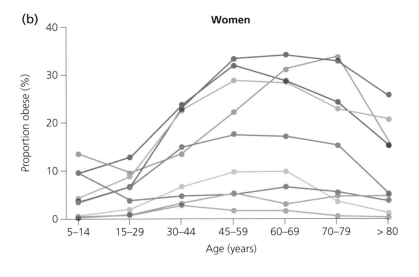

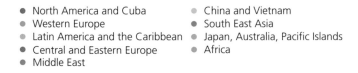

Figure 1.1 Prevalence of obesity worldwide by age and sex. Reprinted from Haslam and James 2005 with permission from Elsevier.

TABLE 1.1

Prevalence of obesity, defined by waist circumference,* in men and women in Europe and the USA

	Men (%)	Women (%)
USA[1]	36.9	55.1
Spain[2]	30.5	37.8
Italy[3]	24.0	37.0
UK[4]	29.0	26.0
The Netherlands[5]	14.8	21.0
Germany[6]	20.0	20.5

*High waist circumference: ≥ 102 cm in men or ≥ 88 cm in women, except in Germany (≥ 103 cm and ≥ 92 cm, respectively).
[1]Ford S et al. *Obes Res* 2003;11:1223–31; [2]Alvarez Leon EE et al. *Med Clin (Barc)* 2003;120:172–4; [3]OECI. *Ital Heart J* 2004;5(suppl 3):49–92; [4]Rushton D et al. *National Diet and Nutrition Survey*, vol. 4. London: ONS, 2004; [5]Visscher TLS et al. *Int J Obes* 2004;28:1309–16; [6]Liese AD et al. *Eur J Nutr* 2001;40:282–8.

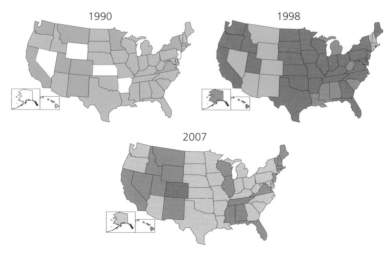

1990   1998   2007

☐ No data ■ <10% ■ 10–14% ■ 15–19% ■ 20–24% ■ 25–29% ■ ≥30%

Figure 1.2 Obesity trends among US adults (obesity is defined as body mass index ≥ 30 kg/m², or about 30 lb [13 kg] overweight for a 5'4" [163 cm] person). Reproduced from the Behavioral Risk Factor Surveillance System, Centers for Disease Control. www.cdc.gov/nccdphp/dnpa/obesity/trend/maps

The maps in Figure 1.3 illustrate the rising levels of obesity throughout Europe over the past decade, demonstrating a widespread problem; this is particularly severe in some southern European countries.

Projections by the World Health Organization indicate that by 2015 approximately 2.3 billion adults worldwide will be overweight and more than 700 million will be obese.

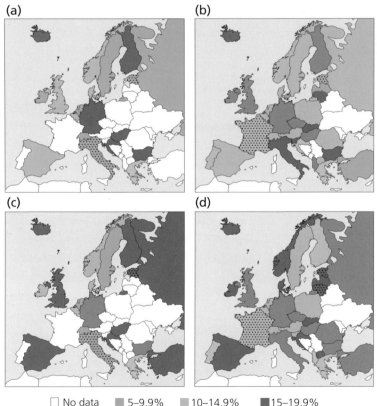

Figure 1.3 Prevalence of obesity in Europe, in men in (a) 1990–1994 and (b) 2000–2005, and in women in (c) 1990–1994 and (d) 2000–2005. The maps show the rapid increase in prevalence in both men and women, and the higher prevalence overall in women than men. © International Obesity Task Force, 2005.

Childhood obesity

Childhood obesity is also increasing rapidly in prevalence worldwide, and has already reached epidemic proportions in some areas. According to the US Surgeon General's call to action, the number of overweight children in the USA has doubled since 1980 and the number of overweight adolescents has trebled. However, recent data from Western Europe, the UK and Australia suggest that a plateau may have been reached.

The prevalence of obesity is increasing rapidly in developing countries, following the trend established in westernized economies. For example, in Thailand the prevalence of obesity in children aged 5–12 years rose from 12.2% to 15.6% in just 2 years.

Childhood obesity is discussed in more detail in Chapter 10.

Burden on general health

Excess bodyweight is the sixth most important risk factor contributing to the overall burden of disease worldwide. As well as being a disease in its own right, obesity is a key risk factor for serious chronic conditions, particularly diabetes, cardiovascular disease and many forms of cancer. (The consequences of obesity are discussed in detail in Chapters 4 and 5.)

Analyses carried out for the 2002 World Health Report indicate that approximately 58% of cases of diabetes, 21% of ischemic heart disease and 8–42% of certain cancers globally were attributable to a BMI above 21 kg/m^2. The International Obesity Task Force (IOTF) reports that 1.7 billion of the world's population is already at a heightened risk of weight-related non-communicable diseases such as type 2 diabetes. Figure 1.4 shows the alarming levels of diabetes secondary to the obesity epidemic in the USA.

Obesity also leads to a plethora of non-fatal but debilitating health problems: respiratory difficulties, chronic musculoskeletal problems such as osteoarthritis, skin problems and infertility. These are discussed in more detail in Chapter 5.

Figure 1.5 demonstrates the years of ill health and lives lost between 30 and 75 years of age due to excess bodyweight, based on estimates of the prevalence of obesity-related disorders and the

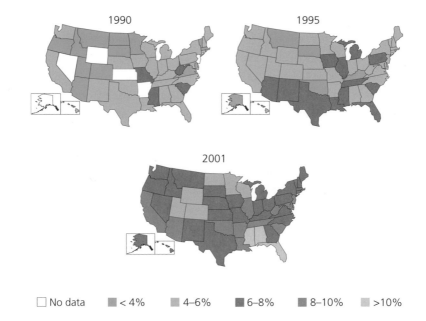

□ No data   ■ < 4%   ■ 4–6%   ■ 6–8%   ■ 8–10%   ■ >10%

Figure 1.4 Prevalence of diabetes among US adults. Reproduced from the Behavioral Risk Factor Surveillance System, Centers for Disease Control. www.cdc.gov/nccdphp/dnpa/obesity/trend/maps

number of deaths as a result, along with the prevalence of raised BMI according to age, and the proportion of the disease burden attributable to excess weight. The patterns show the domination of diabetes and cardiovascular disease as well as the various different cancers linked with obesity. The burden of disease is particularly marked in Central and Eastern Europe.

The number of deaths per year attributable to obesity is roughly 30 000 in the UK and ten times that in the USA.

Even if prevention of obesity in England were 100% successful with immediate effect, and not one single person gained any more weight, there are already enough obese individuals to make an epidemic of diabetes inevitable. Clearly, therefore, treatment of obesity is as important as prevention.

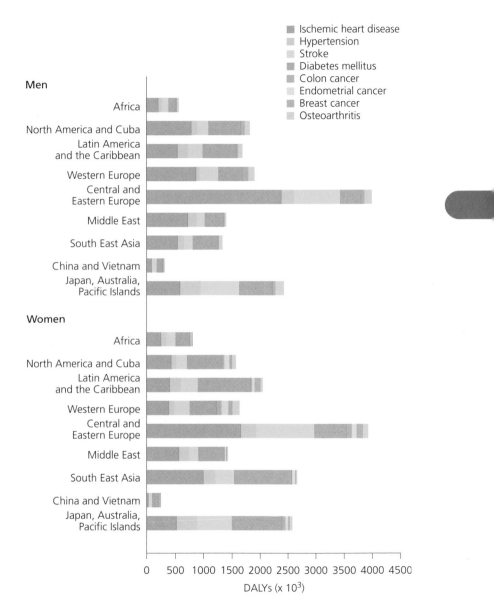

Figure 1.5 Disability-adjusted life-years (DALYs) lost due to obesity in men and women worldwide. Reprinted from Haslam and James 2005 with permission from Elsevier.

Key points – epidemiology

- Obesity has reached epidemic proportions worldwide.
- The situation in the UK will be as bad as that in the USA within a decade if nothing is done.
- Obesity is a key risk factor for serious chronic conditions, particularly diabetes, cardiovascular disease and many forms of cancer.
- Obesity also leads to a plethora of non-fatal but debilitating health problems.
- Management of obesity is synonymous with prevention of cardiometabolic disease, and must be a priority.
- Treatment of obesity is intervention too late; prevention is vital to protect the long-term health of patients.

Key references

Allison DB, Fontaine KR, Manson JE et al. Annual deaths attributable to obesity in the United States. *JAMA* 1999;282:1530–8.

Ezzati M, Lopez AD, Rodgers A et al; Comparative Risk Assessment Collaborating Group. Selected major risk factors and global and regional burden of disease. *Lancet* 2002; 360:1347–60.

Haslam DW, James WP. Obesity. *Lancet* 2005;366:1197–209.

James WPT, Jackson-Leach R, Ni Mhurchu C et al. Overweight and obesity (high body mass index). In: Ezzati M, Lopez AD, Rodgers A, Murray CJL, eds. *Comparative Quantification of Health Risks: Global and Regional Burden of Disease Attributable to Selected Major Risk Factors*, vol 1. Geneva: WHO, 2004:497–596. www.who.int/publications/cra/chapters/volume1/0497-0596.pdf

National Statistics. *Health Survey for England 2003*. Joint Health Surveys Unit. London: The Stationery Office, 2004. www.dh.gov.uk/en/Publicationsand Statistics/Publications/Publications Statistics/DH_4098712

Scottish Health Survey – 2003 results.
www.scotland.gov.uk/Publications/2005/11/25145024/50251

US Public Health Service. *The Surgeon General's call to action to prevent and decrease overweight and obesity 2001.* Rockville, MD: US Department of Health and Human Services, 2001.
www.surgeongeneral.gov/topics/obesity/calltoaction/CalltoAction.pdf

WHO. *Global Strategy on Diet, Physical Activity and Health.*
www.who.int/dietphysicalactivity/publications/facts/obesity/en

WHO. *Media Centre fact sheet: obesity and overweight.*
www.who.int/mediacentre/factsheets/fs311/en/index.html

Not to broach the subject of excess weight with a patient is a dereliction of duty as a health professional. The initial approach taken is crucial, however, as an individual can be permanently engaged or alienated depending on the opening gambit.

Patients who smoke are rapidly identified for intervention, and the same should be true of anyone who is obese. If a patient attending with an unrelated disorder is clearly obese, asking after their general health is a useful prologue to measurement of blood pressure, weight and blood lipid profile and opens the door for more extensive assessment and intervention at a later date. A patient attending a diabetes or cardiovascular clinic can be asked whether they have lost or gained weight recently. Any patient can be offered a 'well patient check' during a consultation, which will include measurement of weight and waist circumference. 'Best practice in weight management' can be performed in the last 2 minutes of any consultation, provided that appropriate follow-up is offered. These 2 minutes are the most important part of the entire weight-loss program.

Assessment of body fat

It is the distribution of fat, not just its presence, that is crucial in determining cardiometabolic risk. Moreover, the presence of a large and regularly exercised muscle mass confers considerable protection from the effects of excess body fat. Thus, as well as being as accurate as possible and appropriate for widespread use in a clinical context, the ideal measure should take body morphology into account.

Body mass index, calculated as weight in kg divided by square of height in meters (kg/m^2), is in widespread use as a measure of adiposity (Table 2.1). It is a useful statistical tool for population and epidemiological studies, and is arguably still the most valuable measure of overweight and obesity in children. For individual adults, however, BMI can be misleading, and it is inaccurate as a predictor of disease.

TABLE 2.1

Body mass index (BMI) and waist circumference as measures of adiposity

	BMI (kg/m^2)	Waist circumference (cm)	
		Men	Women
Definition of obesity for Caucasians			
Not overweight	< 25.0	< 94.0	< 80.0
Overweight–pre-obese	25.0–29.9	94.0–101.9	80.0–87.9
Overweight–obese	≥ 30.0	≥ 102.0	≥ 88.0
Definition of normal weight in Asians			
	18.5–23.0	< 85	< 80

BMI is a crude measure of a person's size and fails to differentiate between the various body morphologies that confer varying degrees of risk, and it may be accounted for by a high lean body mass. Fat carried within the abdomen (visceral fat) is metabolically active and a major predictor of risk, whereas peripheral, subcutaneous or gluteal fat is relatively inert. Highly trained athletes such as rugby players and American football players are often-cited examples of misidentified obesity: their massive shoulders but slim waists often result in a BMI greater than 30 kg/m^2, although they carry little fat. Table 2.2 demonstrates how BMI varies with similar percentage body fat from 20.4 for Ethiopians to 29.5 for Polynesians This also serves to highlight the importance of ethnic-specific criteria for assessment of obesity and associated risk.

The true victim of flawed biometric analysis, however, is the individual with skinny legs and arms but a pot belly who is at high risk of cardiovascular disease. These individuals have a 'normal' BMI despite a high fat mass and may therefore escape identification and slip through the clinical net. These individuals are also at high risk for frailty and disability with increasing age. Thus, BMI is not the ideal measure for clinical practice, and is not suitable as a self-assessment tool as it involves two measurements and a calculation.

TABLE 2.2

Body mass index (BMI) in different races at a constant body fat percentage

Race	Overweight BMI
White	25.0
Black	26.3
Chinese	23.1
Thai	22.1
Ethiopian	20.4
Indonesian	21.8
Polynesian	29.5

Waist circumference is directly proportional to the amount of visceral fat and is therefore an accurate marker of cardiometabolic risk. Correct measurement is shown in Figure 2.1. Measurements are reproducible with little practice and provide a tangible figure: 40 inches (102 cm) is a meaningful term compared with the abstract score of BMI. Patients can easily measure waist circumference themselves.

Waist circumference is gaining recognition as a more accurate indicator of cardiometabolic risk than BMI, and is being increasingly embraced in routine medical practice. Definitions of overweight and obesity in terms of waist circumference are given in Table 2.1. A degree of abdominal obesity is usually recognizable as soon as a patient enters the clinic, and may well represent potentially serious underlying pathology that requires identification and management. Even if the patient's BMI is normal, the clinician has a responsibility to undertake appropriate risk management. Measurement of blood pressure and evaluation of the blood lipid profile and blood glucose is mandatory in such individuals.

Waist circumference is also a useful and tangible marker of weight loss (or gain) for patients. An individual who has increased their physical activity and maintained their dietary intake will lose centimeters around the waist even though they may gain weight as muscle mass increases. Monitoring waist circumference will therefore

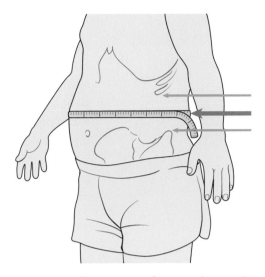

Figure 2.1 Measurement of waist circumference. The tape is set around the waist at a level midway (pink arrow) between the lower rib and the iliac crest (blue arrows), at about the level of the umbilicus (not the belt line). The patient should have fully exhaled, without forcing, with the abdomen relaxed. The measurement should be read from the side, not at the front. The patient can assist by passing the tape behind their own back to avoid over-familiarity and inappropriate physical contact. Classification of obesity by waist circumference is shown in Table 2.1.

keep them motivated when lack of change in bodyweight might prove demoralizing.

Certain ethnic groups, particularly those of South Asian origin, are inherently at higher risk of comorbid disease at smaller waist circumferences. Guidelines such as the International Diabetes Federation's metabolic syndrome criteria have lowered the threshold of abdominal circumference for these groups to reflect the increased likelihood of cardiometabolic disease (see Table 4.1, page 39).

Waist:hip ratio (WHR) is another method commonly used in research as a more accurate assessor of risk in an individual than BMI (Figure 2.2). Measurement is unnecessary for routine clinical practice, and it is not suitable as a self-assessment tool as it involves two

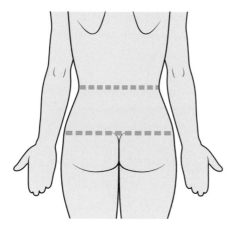

Figure 2.2 Measurement of waist:hip ratio. The waist is measured at the narrowest point and the hips at the widest point, and the ratio of the two calculated. Target values are less than 0.95 for men and less than 0.85 for women.

measurements and a calculation. In the elderly, the hip measurement provides some adjustment for lean body mass.

Bioimpedance analysis (BIA). Although BMI and waist circumference are widely used and easily accommodated within standard clinical practice, other measures of body fat, in particular BIA, are gaining prominence. BIA gives additional information over and above simple biometric measures, by assessing body composition. It involves passing a small electrical current through the body and monitoring the impedance to its flow. Fat increases the resistance, hence the lean:fat ratio can be calculated. This measure can be motivational in patients who become more active and improve their body composition without actually losing weight. It can be assessed using relatively inexpensive stand-on scales and is appropriate for use in obesity clinics, or by patients in their own homes.

Other assessments. Other purely research techniques used to estimate the mass of lean tissue include dual-energy X-ray absorptiometry (DEXA), CT, echo-MRI, densitometry by underwater weighing, natural radioactive potassium (^{40}K) content, and use of isotopic (tritiated or deuterated water) or chemical tracers that provide estimates of total body water from which fat content can be assessed indirectly.

Predicting risk

Waist circumference is a better predictor of risk of cardiometabolic disease (cardiovascular disease, type 2 diabetes) than BMI. Some studies have shown that, after adjustment for waist circumference, a higher BMI appears to protect against cardiometabolic disease, most likely because of a higher skeletal muscle mass, although the presence of relatively more subcutaneous than visceral fat may also be a factor. Other studies have demonstrated that BMI is a much less accurate indicator of risk than WHR or waist circumference, for instance in type 2 diabetes. WHR of 0.85 or less is associated with a low risk compared with WHR of 1 or more, irrespective of BMI.

Taking an accurate history

A full history includes:

- clinical history of diabetes, heart disease and other related illnesses, including depression
- direct questioning for symptoms of cardiometabolic illness or other obesity-related disease, such as polyuria, polydipsia, chest pain, breathlessness, shortness of breath or swelling of the ankles
- family history of excess weight and related illnesses (diabetes, heart disease, cancer)
- social history, including smoking and alcohol intake, support network and employment
- gestation period, birth weight and any neonatal problems
- history of weight gain and perceived underlying causes
- history of weight-loss attempts, successful or otherwise, including diets, exercise regimens and drugs
- current medication, focusing attention on drugs that cause weight gain, particularly insulin, oral hypoglycemic agents, steroids, antipsychotics and antidepressants (see Table 3.2, page 35)
- details of current diet, including a food diary, and an assessment of any abnormal relationship with food, such as emotional eating or binge eating that may need more specific treatment
- physical activity – both routine daily and leisure time – and reasons for restrictions.

Physical examination

The examination should include measurement of height, weight and waist circumference. Body fat analysis is optional but is useful for identifying patients with a normal BMI but high percentage of fat and for monitoring progress, in particular providing encouragement to patients who are improving their health by increased activity but who fail to lose weight. A general visual assessment of a person's fat distribution and body morphology is useful to define central, peripheral or mixed pattern of fat distribution. The presence of any dysmorphic features should be noted, as these may suggest the presence of an obesity syndrome.

Measurement of blood pressure is important. Any further examinations are dictated by other symptoms that present. Baseline investigations include measurement of thyroid function, urea and electrolytes, fasting plasma glucose, lipid profile and liver function tests. Other investigations may be appropriate depending on the history and examination or comorbid illness, such as measurement of HbA_{1c} and microalbuminuria in a patient with diabetes, or B-type natriuretic peptide and echocardiogram in a patient with suspected heart failure. The Epworth Sleepiness Score is a simple tool for assessing the likelihood of significant obstructive sleep apnea.

An informal impression might be gained of a patient's level of engagement, based on their reason for attendance and whether they are motivated to lose weight, and the basis for their motivation. It is also important to ascertain the patient's expectations in terms of weight loss and whether these are realistic.

Key points – patient assessment

- The presence of obesity should be acknowledged and tackled, whatever the reason for a patient's presentation.
- The initial approach is crucial: an individual can be permanently engaged or alienated depending on the opening gambit.
- The best initial screening method is to look at the patient: an obese abdomen is a simple physical sign to pick up but can be indicative of potentially serious underlying disease.
- Waist circumference is directly proportional to the amount of visceral fat and is gaining recognition as a more accurate indicator of cardiometabolic risk than body mass index, and is being increasingly embraced in routine medical practice.
- Decreased waist circumference in the absence of weight loss can keep a patient motivated.

Key references

Balkau B, Deanfield JE, Després JP et al. International Day for the Evaluation of Abdominal Obesity (IDEA): a study of waist circumference, cardiovascular disease, and diabetes mellitus in 168,000 primary care patients in 63 countries. *Circulation* 2007;116:1942–51.

Clark NG, Fox KM, Grand S; SHIELD study group. Symptoms of diabetes and their association with the risk and presence of diabetes: findings from the Study to Help Improve Early evaluation and management of risk factors Leading to Diabetes (SHIELD). *Diabetes Care* 2007;30:2868–73.

Han TS, Sattar N, Lean M. ABC of obesity. Assessment of obesity and its clinical implications. *BMJ* 2006;333:695–8.

Wang Y, Rimm EB, Stampfer MJ et al. Comparison of abdominal adiposity and overall obesity in predicting risk of type 2 diabetes among men. *Am J Clin Nutr* 2005;81:555–63.

Evolution

For our prehistoric ancestors, the rules for survival were simple: eat whenever possible, and rest to conserve energy for times when it was needed to preserve life. Those endowed with the so-called 'thrifty gene' (although no such individual gene exists) could store energy efficiently as fat, thus thriving when food was available and surviving times of fast and famine.

The environment has evolved rapidly since then, however, without any evolutionary process in humans to compensate. Natural selection now favors different groups: those with the thrifty gene are genetically predisposed to suffer premature death; eating for survival and conserving vital energy have transformed into overeating and underactivity, conspiring to cause serious chronic disease.

Regulation of energy balance and fat mass

Fat mass is maintained relatively constant on a day-to-day and week-to-week basis. A physiological system monitors fat mass and regulates energy balance via nutritional, endocrine and neural signals, coordinated by a neural network in the central nervous system (CNS). CNS efferents modulate the metabolic functions of the liver, skeletal muscle and adipose tissues, as well as pancreatic endocrine function and motor and secretory functions of the gut.

Alteration in stable weight by forced overfeeding or food deprivation induces physiological changes that resist these perturbations: with weight loss, appetite increases and energy expenditure falls; with overfeeding, appetite decreases and energy expenditure elevates. Thus we are adapted to facilitating the storage of energy in fat depots.

Given the nature and complexity of the system, it is not hard to appreciate how complex inherited genetic polymorphisms can lead to variations in fat mass – to which the genetic contribution is almost 70%. It is also the nature of this system that makes the failure of 'dieting' inevitable: a fall in energy intake is rapidly detected, leading to hunger and reduced energy expenditure. As fat mass decreases, the neural networks that regulate energy balance ensure that fat mass returns to the previous level. Although the two sides of the energy balance equation – energy intake and storage versus energy expenditure – are integrated, it is useful conceptually to consider each separately.

Energy storage

Food is digested to the basic nutrients – glucose, amino acids and fatty acids. Glucose and amino acids provide 4 kcal energy per gram; fatty acids provide 9 kcal/g. Alcohol provides 7 kcal/g and is an obligatory nutrient, which means that the only pathway for disposal is oxidation for energy. Therefore, food eaten concomitantly that is in excess of energy requirement will be stored as fat.

Regulation of energy intake

This system has three components:
- an afferent system
- a central integrating system
- an efferent system.

Afferent system. Small decreases in plasma glucose can trigger hunger but increases in plasma nutrient levels are probably not directly important in the regulation of appetite.

Adipose tissue. Leptin secreted by adipocytes provides a signal to the brain to indicate the amount of fat stored in adipose tissue. Leptin acts at the arcuate nucleus of the hypothalamus to suppress neuropeptide Y (NPY)/AgRP, which increases food intake, and to stimulate proopiomelanocortin (POMC), which decreases food intake. Leptin also has peripheral metabolic effects that promote energy utilization. The regulatory systems are exquisitely sensitive to a fall in plasma leptin levels, which occur in response to caloric restriction even before a decrease in fat mass.

Stomach. The presence or absence of food in the stomach and the state of energy balance affect both the motor and secretory functions of the stomach. Gastric distension, antral diameter and pyloric tone mediate satiation in the setting of nutrient absorption from the

proximal gut. The hormone ghrelin, which increases hunger, is secreted
by the oxyntic glands in the stomach mucosa when empty; levels rise
sharply before every meal and fall promptly when the stomach is full.

Intestine. The presence of glucose, fatty acids and amino acids in
the gut:

- induce the release of peptides, such as cholecystokinin (CCK),
  glucagon-like peptide-1 (GLP-1) and peptide YY (PYY), which
  integrate behavioral aspects of food intake, digestion and gut
  motility, insulin production by the pancreas, and intermediary
  metabolism in the liver, adipose tissue and skeletal muscle
- activate vagal afferents that convey information to integrating
  centers in the brainstem and hypothalamus.

Central integrating system. The humeral, neural and metabolic signals
act by influencing the expression and release of various peptide
neurotransmitters in the arcuate nucleus. Vagal afferents project to the
nucleus of the tractus solitarius, which 'switches' information between
the hypothalamic circuits and vagal efferents. Output from the arcuate
nucleus is predominantly to the paraventricular nucleus (PVN) and
lateral hypothalamic nucleus. Serotonergic, catecholaminergic,
dopaminergic, endocannabinoid and opioidergic pathways integrate the
centers that regulate food intake and feeding behavior with the centers
responsible for motor function, emotion, reward, reproduction and
sleep.

Effector system. Outputs from the PVN participate in the regulation of
autonomic function and permit neuroendocrine responses that are
appropriate to the state of energy balance, such as a decrease in thyroid
and gonadal function in states of starvation or marked energy
imbalance.

The perifornical and lateral hypothalamic areas (LHA), stimulation
of which increases food intake, integrate information from the arcuate
nucleus, vagal and visceral sensory inputs and brain areas associated
with reward, motivation, learning and memory. Outputs to the cortex,
limbic system and thalamus integrate a range of behaviors and emotions
critical to the safe and effective procurement of food. Outputs from the

brainstem and spinal cord regulate chewing, swallowing and movement, and autonomic control of brown and white adipose tissue, pancreas, gastrointestinal tract, liver, muscle and blood vessels.

Regulation of energy expenditure

Total energy expenditure (TEE) is accounted for by three components:

- basal metabolic rate (BMR)
- physical activity level (PAL) (intentional, incidental and non-exercise-associated thermogenesis [NEAT])
- the thermic effect of food (TEF).

Basal metabolic rate reflects the energy expended on the basic metabolic processes necessary for life and constitutes 45–70% of TEE in adults. It can be measured accurately using indirect calorimetry in the morning after 8 hours' rest and 12 hours after a meal, while supine and awake. Calorimetric measurement requires abstinence from strenuous physical activity the day before, a state of mental relaxation and an ambient environmental temperature that does not evoke shivering or sweating. It is therefore perhaps more appropriately termed resting energy expenditure (REE). REE is higher in men than women, and in both sexes it depends on fat-free mass, fat mass and age. Fat-free mass is the best predictor of REE and accounts for most of the interindividual variability; however, a large fat mass will also contribute significantly to REE. It is now also recognized that humans have deposits of active brown adipose tissue that generates heat in cold environments, although the extent to which these deposits affect BMR in thermoneutral environments is uncertain. Various factors may increase REE, including thyroid hormone, growth hormone and activation of the sympathetic nervous system.

Physical activity level. Energy expenditure can vary substantially depending on the level of habitual physical activity. The PAL is the energy cost of physical activity, expressed as a multiple of 24-hour BMR. A desirable PAL includes regular physical activity (at work or leisure time) with an intensity and duration that will reduce the

27

risk of becoming overweight and developing a variety of non-communicable chronic diseases that are usually associated as comorbidities with obesity; this corresponds to PAL values of 1.75 and higher. An expert panel of the International Obesity Task Force (IOTF) suggested a lower PAL range of 1.50–1.55 as representative of sedentary individuals. The categories shown in Table 3.1 represent the different levels of activity associated with a population's lifestyle.

Non-exercise associated thermogenesis is often neglected as a component of physical activity. NEAT has a high degree of heritability and may be an important defense against obesity. There appears to be a link between neural circuits that modulate sleep, addiction and the stress response and NEAT.

TABLE 3.1

Classification of lifestyles in relation to the intensity of habitual physical activity or physical activity level (PAL)

Lifestyle category	Characteristics	PAL value
Sedentary or light activity	Occupation does not demand much physical effort Motor vehicles used for transport Does not exercise or participate in sports regularly Leisure time spent mostly sitting or standing relatively still	1.40–1.69
Active or moderately active	Occupation involves regular but not particularly strenuous activity, or regularly spends time each day in moderate-to-vigorous physical activities of necessity or for recreational purposes	1.70–1.99
Vigorous or vigorously active	Engages regularly in strenuous work or in strenuous leisure activities for several hours at a time	2.00–2.40*

*PAL values over 2.40 are difficult to maintain over a long period of time.

Thermic effect of food. The increase in energy expenditure following food intake is a physiological determinant of total daily energy expenditure, accounting for about 10% of the total. Protein intake increases the TEF to a greater extent than equivalent amounts of carbohydrate or fat. The satiating effect of carbohydrate appears to be reduced in obese compared with lean individuals.

Approximately 40% of TEF is believed to be mediated by activation of the sympathetic nervous system. TEF decreases with weight loss – an effect that persists in the post-obese state, thereby promoting weight regain.

The 'obesogenic' environment

Maintenance of a steady bodyweight demands that energy intake matches energy expenditure. A landmark paper published in the *BMJ* in 1995 entitled 'Obesity in Britain: gluttony or sloth?' concluded that reduction in physical activity, rather than increased energy intake, has been the fundamental cause of the current obesity epidemic. A decline in activity was possibly the major feature of the early rise in obesity levels in the 1960s to 1980s. Certainly, the ready availability of labor-saving devices and technology has contributed to this, as have more sedentary occupations, and leisure time based around sedentary activities such as watching television and online/computer-based activities.

Current thinking, however, is that transformation of our food habits has been the major amplifier of the high prevalence of obesity and diabetes, largely in response to intense industry competition. Processing of food is now common but profoundly alters nutritional balance, increases energy density and potentially creates exposure to chemicals of various sorts. Also, food is available day and night in supermarkets and fast-food outlets at almost any geographic location, and in bigger, cheaper and unhealthier portions than ever.

National epidemiological studies have shown that energy intake is now the dominant determinant of weight gain, and in some cases lower physical activity follows rather than precedes weight gain. Critics also point to the well-recognized phenomenon of under-reporting of food intake, especially of food consumed outside the home, as a confounding factor.

A recent paper concurred with the argument that increased food intake is to blame, by comparing the energy expenditure of humans to that of wild mammals, in an attempt to show that humans still perform the amount of physical activity dictated by our natural surroundings. It concluded that physical activity expenditure has not declined over the same period that obesity rates have increased dramatically, and daily energy expenditure of modern man is in line with energy expenditure in wild mammals. It is therefore unlikely that decreased energy expenditure has fuelled the obesity epidemic.

Whichever case is true, the modern 'toxic' or 'obesogenic' environment is conducive to weight gain.

Genetic predisposition

Obesity-related disease is high in Eastern Europe and Latin America, and Asian countries have a disproportionately high burden of disease despite lower obesity rates, reflecting a preponderance of abdominal obesity and proneness to diabetes. This is thought to be due to an underlying genetic predisposition, and becomes apparent on exposure to unhealthy diets and lifestyles.

'Obesity genes'. Genetic factors can determine whether a person is prone to gaining weight, and the likely magnitude of the weight gain, as shown by overfeeding studies in twins. It is estimated that 50–70% of the variation in fat mass between individuals has a genetic basis, due to polygenic environmental interactions rather than individual 'obesity genes'.

Differences in muscle mass and function, spontaneous physical activity, twitchiness and fidgeting, BMR and eating behavior all have varying degrees of heritability from the contributions of many different genes.

Individual 'obesity genes' are described periodically in the scientific press, but each has little relevance in the clinician's struggle against obesity. For example, monogenic mutations that affect leptin secretion, the leptin receptor or the melanocortins are rare and merely represent a footnote in the evaluation of the obesity epidemic.

Environmental factors

Certain groups, such as the Pima Indians of South Dakota and the Nauru islanders in the South Pacific, have suffered from the change in their native environment, whereas other groups have succumbed to environmental pressures following migration. For example, second-generation offspring of migrants to the UK are likely to adopt British patterns of food consumption, increasing dietary fat and reducing fruit and vegetable intake. Indian immigrants have been shown to suffer increased levels of weight gain and obesity after entering the UK, and African American women have higher fat intake and less physical activity than their white counterparts. The nature of the built environment may also be an important factor in limiting both physical activity and food choice.

Life stage

An individual is particularly susceptible to weight gain and weight-related complications at various significant stages of life.

Prenatal/postnatal. Poor maternal nutrition adversely imprints the fetal metabolism, conferring permanent effects on later growth, body shape, fatness and energy regulation of the child. Breastfeeding may protect both mother and child from obesity, but breastfeeding rates are poor in developed countries, particularly in the UK where the prevalence and duration of breastfeeding are amongst the lowest in Europe.

New growth charts were introduced in England and Wales in May 2009 that are based on data collected by the World Health Organization from breastfed babies. These charts take into account the normal slowing of weight gain in breastfed babies at around 8 weeks. In the past this has been misinterpreted as 'failure to thrive' and mothers have been encouraged to 'top up' with formula feed in order to maintain growth along a given centile on a chart, a practice that is misguided and can lay the foundations for childhood obesity.

Childhood. Rapid growth in children aged between 5 and 7 years can occur as a result of 'adiposity rebound' – a period of increasing growth and BMI that may coincide with exposure to new environments and

31

food and activity behavior patterns; an early adiposity rebound may lead to increased risk of obesity later in life. The causes and issues relating to obesity in children are discussed in Chapter 10.

Adolescence also represents a time of increased autonomy and changing behavioral patterns – irregular meals, changed food habits and prolonged periods of inactivity, combined with physiological changes that promote increased fat deposition, particularly in girls.

Early adulthood, for women in particular, can induce significant weight gain; the contraceptive pill and/or pregnancy can be a stimulus for weight gain. Co-habiting and meal sharing with a partner may also lead to increased energy consumption. Repeated pregnancies may also induce long-term weight gain.

Midlife. In women, menopause tends to be associated with weight gain, particularly around the abdomen. Hormonal changes and decreased physical activity may be responsible, although the exact process is not fully understood. In men, reduction of leisure and work activity and the adoption of more sedentary lifestyles are important factors in weight gain.

Old age. The elderly have unique risk factors, as they tend to suffer from sarcopenic obesity – a reduction in muscle mass alongside an increased amount of body fat. The causes and issues relating to obesity in the elderly are discussed in Chapter 10.

Socioeconomic status

In developed countries, increased levels of deprivation are linked with obesity. In England, 18.7% of managerial and professional women are classified as obese, compared with 29.1% of women in less prestigious occupations. The most easily affordable foods are usually higher in fat and energy density, compounded by the fact that those with fewer financial resources may spend more time in sedentary activities, such as watching television.

In the developed world, disadvantage is associated with:
- lower consumption of healthier food options; compared with higher social groups, lower social groups have lower intake of fruit and vegetables, protein, fiber and many vitamins and minerals
- poor access to sports facilities
- less physical activity outside work and less participation in sport.

In developed countries, obesity used to be linked with wealth, but in the 21st century it is closely linked with deprivation. For example, in the USA, low-income families have a higher level of obesity; in China, there is an even split between lower and higher income families, with an intermediate level in middle-income families.

Earlier lifestyle

Recidivism among those who lose weight by any method other than bariatric surgery is well recognized, and adults who have previously been overweight and have lost weight are at an increased risk of becoming obese. 'Yo-yo' dieting is dangerous because the cumulative weight gain following recurrent attempts at reducing weight is a risk factor in its own right. People who have quit smoking are also predisposed to weight gain. Individuals who change from an active to an inactive or sedentary lifestyle are inevitably at risk of becoming overweight/obese.

Other factors

Sleep restriction and obstructive sleep apnea (OSA). Sleep restriction in both children and adults has been associated with a predisposition to obesity. Obesity and type 2 diabetes are also more common in shift workers. OSA, which is becoming increasingly common, is associated with not only obesity and type 2 diabetes but also with hypertension and a substantial increase in the risk of cardiovascular events.

Psychosocial stress. Data from both animal and human studies have demonstrated a relationship between perception of psychosocial stress and obesity.

Medical conditions

Some medical conditions such as Cushing's disease and hypothyroidism predispose patients to obesity. Cushing's disease has characteristic features that should be looked for. Hypothyroidism seldom leads to significant weight gain but makes weight loss more difficult. Damage to the hypothalamus from neoplasms, infiltrations or other pathological processes, surgery or accidental trauma can lead to hyperphagia, abnormal eating behaviors and weight gain. A number of congenital conditions due to chromosomal disorders, for example Prader–Willi syndrome, Down syndrome and, in incredibly rare instances, monogenetic conditions such as leptin deficiency are associated with obesity.

Psychiatric conditions

The prevalence of obesity is approximately 50% higher in people with serious mental health problems than in the general population, reflecting chaotic lifestyles, lack of involvement with traditional healthcare systems and possibly an underlying genetic predisposition to metabolic complications.

The physical health of these patients is a major issue. Self-management is notoriously poor, and many secondary care centers are ill-equipped to manage simple health screening, let alone potentially complex metabolic disorders, whilst primary care practitioners are often uneasy managing mental health problems. The prescribing of antipsychotic agents that cause weight gain not only adds to the metabolic burden for such patients but may reduce self-esteem even further in already psychologically fragile individuals.

Each patient's profile should be assessed on their own merits but their physical health needs must be prioritized; 60% of patients with schizophrenia die prematurely, largely from cardiometabolic complications, but only 10% self-harm. Patients susceptible to weight gain and metabolic sequelae should be considered for medication review, with the possible introduction of more metabolically acceptable agents.

Medicines

Table 3.2 gives an overview of drugs known to cause weight gain, and some 'weight friendly' alternatives. Clinical decisions should balance the benefits of a drug against its propensity for causing side effects, including promotion of excess weight.

TABLE 3.2

Medications that cause weight gain, and 'weight friendly' alternatives

Agents that cause weight gain	'Weight friendly' alternatives
Antipsychotics Most second-generation agents especially olanzapine	Aripiprazole
Antidepressants Tricyclics MAOIs Mirtazapine	SSRIs are largely weight neutral or promote weight loss, although some cause weight gain in some patients
Other psychiatric drugs Lithium Carbamazepine	
Corticosteroids (Promote central accumulation of fat and loss of muscle mass)	
Antihypertensives Beta-blockers (may also restrict physical activity because of fatigue)	ACE inhibitors Angiotensin receptor blockers Calcium channel blockers
Hypoglycemic agents Insulin Thiazolidinediones Sulfonylureas	Metformin DPP-4 inhibitors (e.g. sitagliptin, vildagliptin) are weight neutral GLP mimetics (exenatide and liraglutide) may promote weight loss

CONTINUED

TABLE 3.2 (CONTINUED)

Agents that cause weight gain	'Weight friendly' alternatives
Oral contraceptives Progesterogenic compounds	
Anticonvulsants	
Carbamazepine	Topirimate
Phenytoin	Zonisamide
Sodium valproate	
Others	
Pizotifen (migraine prophylaxis)	
Pregabalin (neuropathic pain)	
Gabapentin (neuropathic pain)	

ACE, angiotensin-converting enzyme; DPP, dipeptidyl peptidase; GLP, glucagon-like peptide; MAOI, monoamine oxidase inhibitor; SSRI, selective serotonin-reuptake inhibitor.

Key points – causes and science

- Physiological and genetic influences that promoted survival of our ancestors are now conspiring against us to promote obesity and comorbid disease.
- Genetic influences act alongside environmental factors to promote obesity.
- Most causes of adult obesity are within the grasp of an individual to control, but babies and children rely on their parents and carers to provide an appropriate environment.
- Iatrogenic causes of obesity should be considered. The effect on weight of managing comorbid conditions is important, particularly diabetes in which weight gain is potentially catastrophic.

Key references

Anon. Gene-nutrition and gene-physical activity interactions in the etiology of obesity workshop. *Obesity (Silver Spring)* 2008;16(Suppl 3): S1–96.

Department of Health. *Health survey for England – trends*. London: Department of Health, 2005.

Eisenmann JC. Insight into the causes of the recent secular trend in pediatric obesity: common sense does not always prevail for complex, multi-factorial phenotypes. *Prev Med* 2006;42:329–35.

Erlichman J, Kerbey A, James P. Are current physical activity guidelines adequate to prevent unhealthy weight gain? *A scientific appraisal for consideration by an Expert Panel of the International Obesity Task Force (IOTF)*. London: IOTF, 2001:113.

Friedman JM. Obesity: causes and control of excess body fat. *Nature* 2009;459:340–2.

Haslam DW, James WP. Obesity. *Lancet* 2005;366:1197–209.

Landman J, Cruickshank JK. A review of ethnicity, health and nutrition-related diseases in relation to migration in the United Kingdom. *Public Health Nutr* 2001;4:647–57.

Lenard NR, Berthoud HR. Central and peripheral regulation of food intake and physical activity: pathways and genes. *Obesity (Silver Spring)* 2008;16(Suppl 3):S11–22.

McKeigue PM, Shah B, Marmot MG. Relation of central obesity and insulin resistance with high diabetes prevalence and cardiovascular risk in South Asians. *Lancet* 1991;337:382–6.

Monteiro PO, Victora CG. Rapid growth in infancy and childhood and obesity in later life – a systematic review. *Obes Rev* 2005;6:143–54.

Must A, Jacques PF, Dallal GE et al. Long-term morbidity and mortality of overweight adolescents: a follow up of the Harvard Growth Study of 1922 to 1935. *N Engl J Med* 1992;327:1350–5.

Novak CM, Levine JA. Central neural and endocrine mechanisms of non-exercise activity thermogenesis and their potential impact on obesity. *J Neuroendocrinol* 2007;19:923–40.

Prentice AM, Jebb SA. Obesity in Britain: gluttony or sloth? *BMJ* 1995;311:437–9.

Saris WH, Blair SN, van Baak MA et al. How much physical activity is enough to prevent unhealthy weight gain? Outcome of the IASO 1st Stock Conference and consensus statement. *Obes Rev* 2003;4:101–14.

Walcott-McQuigg JA. The relationship between stress and weight-control behavior in African-American women. *J Natl Med Assoc* 1995;87:427–32.

Williamson DF, Madans J, Pamuk E et al. A prospective study of childbearing and 10-year weight gain in US white women 25 to 45 years of age. *Int J Obes Relat Metab Disord* 1994;18:561–9.

Overweight/obesity as a whole predisposes to, or is associated with, numerous cardiac complications such as coronary heart disease (CHD), heart failure and sudden cardiac death as a result of abnormalities in blood glucose, lipids, blood pressure, coagulation and inflammation. Independent of any of the other known cardiometabolic risk factors, obesity is associated with hypertension, tachycardia, left ventricular hypertrophy, increased collagen deposition, reduced cardiac contractility and increased end-diastolic pressure. The major circulatory complications are increased total and pulmonary blood volume, high cardiac output and elevated left ventricular end-diastolic pressure.

Metabolic syndrome

'Metabolic syndrome' describes the clustering in an individual of the most dangerous risk factors for myocardial infarction, namely poor glycemic control, abdominal obesity (Figure 4.1), dyslipidemia and hypertension.

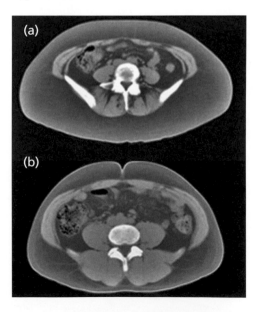

Figure 4.1 CT scans showing cross-sections of the abdomens of two individuals. In (a) the fat is predominantly located subcutaneously. In (b) a large amount of fat is present in the omentum and around the viscera.

The International Diabetes Federation (IDF) updated the definition of metabolic syndrome in 2005, making abdominal obesity a requirement for a diagnosis of the metabolic syndrome, and providing different obesity cut-off points for different ethnic groups. This definition takes account of the fact that central adiposity is common to each component of the metabolic syndrome. The criteria are summarized in Table 4.1.

TABLE 4.1

International Diabetes Federation definition of the metabolic syndrome

A person must have:

Central obesity (waist circumference ≥ 94 cm for Europid men and ≥ 80 cm for Europid women)

plus any *two* of the following four factors:

- **raised TG level**: ≥ 150 mg/dL (1.7 mmol/L), or specific treatment for this lipid abnormality
- **reduced HDL cholesterol**: < 40 mg/dL (1.03 mmol/L) in men and < 50 mg/dL (1.29 mmol/L) in women, or specific treatment for this lipid abnormality
- **raised blood pressure**: systolic BP ≥ 130 or diastolic BP ≥ 85 mmHg, or treatment of previously diagnosed hypertension
- **raised fasting plasma glucose** ≥ 100 mg/dL (5.6 mmol/L), or previously diagnosed type 2 diabetes

Waist circumference for South Asians/Chinese/Japanese

Male	*≥ 90 cm*
Female	*≥ 80 cm*

For ethnic South and Central Americans use South Asian data until more specific data are available. For Sub-Saharan Africans, Eastern Mediterranean and Middle East (Arab) populations use Europid data until more specific data are available.

BP, blood pressure; HDL, high-density lipoprotein; TG, triglyceride.

Epidemiology. An estimated 20–30% of middle-aged individuals living in industrialized countries may be affected by the syndrome. As many as 75 million people in the USA alone may exhibit the syndrome by 2010. It is estimated that as few as 30% of adults exhibit none of the major characteristics of metabolic syndrome.

Consequences. Metabolic syndrome is commonly a precursor of type 2 diabetes and cardiovascular disease, as well as many other associated conditions.

Patients with metabolic syndrome are three times more likely to experience a heart attack or stroke than people without the syndrome, and are twice as likely to die as a result. They also have a fivefold greater risk of developing type 2 diabetes, adding to the 230 million cases worldwide.

Definition of the metabolic syndrome is of value because it ensures that any patient with a single cardiovascular risk factor, including obesity, is screened for the others, as their presence is statistically highly likely and coexistent cardiometabolic risks multiply the overall risk. It also ensures that a patient with multiple risk factors, even those considered borderline, is managed as a high-risk individual. The aim of management is to tackle the syndrome as a whole, and obesity in particular. Management of single or even multiple cardiometabolic risk factors, for example hypertension or hyperlipidemia alone, or even the combination of hyperlipidemia, hyperglycemia and hypertension, is insufficient; the fundamental issues of excess and pathologically distributed body fat, exercise deficiency and a nutritionally poor diet require attention.

Not all commentators support the utility of the metabolic syndrome as a concept, and the many published definitions and criteria have served to confuse rather than inform. In addition, many other conditions with shared etiology, such as polycystic ovary syndrome (PCOS; see pages 47–9) and non-alcoholic steatohepatitis (NASH; see pages 58–9), which are characterized by insulin resistance and excess and/or ectopic fat are associated with increased cardiometabolic risk even though the criteria for the metabolic syndrome may not be met.

Insulin resistance is the common denominator for all the risk factors for metabolic syndrome. Insulin, produced by the beta cells of the pancreas, controls the uptake, intracellular utilization and storage of glucose, amino acids and fatty acids, while inhibiting catabolic processes such as the breakdown of glycogen, fat and protein. A major function is to stimulate the uptake of glucose by skeletal muscle, where it is used as a source of energy. Insulin also has separate functions on adipose tissue, where it inhibits lipolysis – the breakdown of triglycerides which releases fatty acids into the bloodstream. Individuals with metabolic syndrome have parallel insulin resistance in both muscles and adipose tissue, so in addition to the high insulin and glucose levels, the concentration of circulating fatty acids and dyslipidemia is also high.

Insulin resistance occurs when the tissues respond sluggishly to its action, causing blood glucose to rise, requiring more insulin to be produced to compensate – hyperinsulinemia. In the early stages of insulin resistance these physiological changes stimulate increased production of insulin, keeping glucose levels under control; with time, however, the feedback mechanisms become disrupted, glucose levels rise and type 2 diabetes ensues.

Effects of insulin resistance on other organs. Only the insulin receptors in liver, muscle and adipose tissue are abnormal in patients with insulin resistance; the other organs of the body have normal sensitivity but become overstimulated because of the high circulating levels of insulin, leading to further complications of metabolic syndrome. The kidneys respond to insulin by retaining salt, which leads to hypertension; 50% of people with high blood pressure have metabolic syndrome. The ability of the kidney to clear uric acid is also compromised, leading to hyperuricemia and gout.

The colon, breast, prostate and other organs are also affected, leading to increased cancer risk (see Chapter 5).

Management. The only logical way to treat one or more of the elements of metabolic syndrome in obese patients is to tackle the insulin resistance, either by weight loss or with specific pharmaco-therapy.

Typically, 10% weight loss will result in:
- 50% reduction in fasting glucose
- 15% reduction in HbA_{1c}
- 8% increase in high-density lipoprotein (HDL)
- 15% reduction in low-density lipoprotein (LDL)
- 30% reduction in triglycerides
- 10 mmHg reduction in systolic and diastolic blood pressure.

Diabetes

The link between obesity and type 2 diabetes is firmly established (Table 4.2; Figure 4.2). The risk of diabetes is magnified in individuals with:
- abdominal rather than peripheral obesity (see Figure 4.1)
- a family history of diabetes
- gestational diabetes (and those whose mothers had gestational diabetes)
- a history of excessive childhood weight gain.

Other factors predisposing to type 2 diabetes mellitus include lack of physical activity, high intake of sugared soft drinks, refined carbohydrate and saturated fat, and low intake of fiber.

TABLE 4.2

The link between obesity and type 2 diabetes

- 90% of individuals who develop type 2 diabetes have BMI > 23 kg/m²
- 80–85% of patients with type 2 diabetes are obese
- 12% of people with BMI > 27 kg/m² have type 2 diabetes
- A man with a waist circumference > 100 cm has a 3.5-fold increased risk of diabetes
- A woman with BMI ≥ 35 kg/m² is over 93 times more likely to develop type 2 diabetes than her lean counterpart
- Each kilogram of weight gained increases the risk of diabetes by 4.5%

BMI, body mass index.

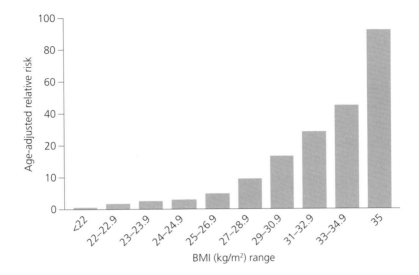

Figure 4.2 Relative risk for type 2 diabetes by body mass index (BMI) in women aged 30–55 years. Data from the Nurses' Health Study 1996.

Individuals of South Asian origin are more at risk from the comorbidities of obesity, including type 2 diabetes, at a lower BMI or waist circumference than their Caucasian counterparts. These ethnic differences are reflected in criteria such as the IDF definition of the metabolic syndrome (see Table 4.1). In Japan, 50% of 70 year olds with BMI $\geq$ 28.0 kg/m² have type 2 diabetes. In some aboriginal communities the rate of diabetes is as high as 33%.

The lag phase between the onset of uncomplicated obesity (BMI > 30 kg/m²) and the development of diabetes can be 10–12 years, although the underlying pathological changes are already developing when the patient is overweight, even though outward signs and symptoms may remain undetected.

Management of obese patients with diabetes

Weight loss. Several major studies, including the Diabetes Prevention Program and the Diabetes Prevention Study, have shown that modest reduction in weight induced by intensive lifestyle modification alone reduces the cumulative incidence of diabetes by 58% (Figure 4.3).

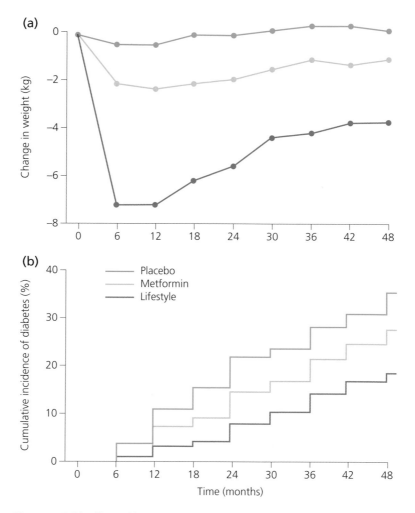

Figure 4.3 (a) Effect of interventions on weight and (b) cumulative incidence of diabetes in the Diabetes Prevention Program. Reproduced with permission from Knowler WC et al. *N Engl J Med* 2002;346:393–403. © Massachusetts Medical Society. All rights reserved.

Weight loss of 0.5–9.0 kg is associated with a 30–40% reduction in diabetes-related mortality.

Patients with diabetes have more difficulty losing weight than those without the condition – given optimum lifestyle advice and support, a diabetic person intent on weight reduction will lose about 50% of that managed by a non-diabetic in a year. However, 5–10% sustainable loss of bodyweight confers massive benefits to the individual: 10% loss of bodyweight equates to a reduction of 30% of the dangerous intra-abdominal fat. Regular and ongoing physical activity and a focus on healthy eating are essential for maintenance of weight loss.

Dietary management. Specific nutritional guidelines apply to obese patients with diabetes. An overall reduction in portion size and energy density is essential, and a regular pattern of meals – breakfast, lunch and dinner – is important; snacking should be avoided. Intake of saturated fat should be very low, and trans fats should be avoided completely. A reduction in overall carbohydrate intake is beneficial in the case of insulin resistance. Carbohydrates consumed should be high in fiber. Sugar and other refined carbohydrates are best avoided or consumed only rarely and in very small quantities. Artificial sweeteners are a reasonable alternative. Carbohydrates with a low glycemic index (GI; see page 73) should be encouraged, as they have a more moderate effect on the postprandial increase in blood glucose. Dietary management of obesity is described in Chapter 6.

Physical activity. Regular physical activity reduces insulin resistance and protects against cardiometabolic disease even if weight is not lost. Both aerobic and resistance activities are beneficial. Physical activity is discussed in more detail in Chapter 7.

Anti-obesity drugs. Specific anti-obesity agents such as orlistat and sibutramine have effects on glucose regulation that are beneficial in the management of diabetes in obese patients. The pharmacotherapy of obesity is discussed in Chapter 9.

Hypoglycemic agents. First-line management of type 2 diabetes in patients with obesity is with metformin (unless contraindicated), which should be initiated at diagnosis, regardless of lifestyle changes that may also be required. The choice of second agent has become less obvious with the introduction of several new agents. Excess weight is the primary etiologic factor behind type 2 diabetes and weight gain can be demoralizing to patients, who are told that weight stability, or preferably loss, is their goal. The oral hypoglycemic agents that induce weight gain (see Table 3.2, page 35) are therefore best avoided.

Metformin. The UK Prospective Diabetes Study (UKPDS) demonstrated metformin to be an effective monotherapy for the treatment of obese patients with diabetes by improving insulin resistance and accordingly reducing plasma insulin and triglyceride levels without risk of hypoglycemia. The absolute reduction in HbA_{1c} was usually 0.6% more than by diet and lifestyle intervention alone. In the UKPDS, micro- and macrovascular complications were reduced by 32% in metformin recipients compared with lifestyle change alone. Metformin is the only oral hypoglycemic agent shown to reduce mortality.

Metformin can cause gastrointestinal upset, although this is minimized by the use of a slow-release formulation. Metformin-induced lactic acidosis is very rare, but for this reason the drug is contraindicated in patients with severe renal impairment or cardiac or hepatic failure.

In the setting of mild-to-moderate renal impairment, a low dose of metformin (maximum of 500 mg twice daily) is generally safe. There is no evidence to support the use of more than 2 g daily, and administration three times daily is not better than twice-daily dosing.

Sulfonylureas have been a traditional mainstay of oral hypoglycemic treatment, alone or in combination with metformin. However, there are concerns that they may advance beta-cell failure and therefore insulin dependency, and possibly reduce survival. During the initial stages of treatment, sulfonylureas induce more impressive reduction in HbA_{1c} than the alternatives, but this effect advantage is short lived.

Thiazolidinediones. The thiazolidinediones rosiglitazone and pioglitazone act as agonists at the peroxisome proliferator-activated nuclear receptor γ and increase insulin sensitivity by activating genes involved in metabolism and fat synthesis. They induce significant improvements in glycemic control but increase body fat and cause weight gain and fluid retention. Adverse effects include heart failure and bone fractures.

Glucosidase inhibitors such as acarbose reduce digestion of starch, slowing the postprandial increase in blood glucose. They are most effective when used in conjunction with other oral hypoglycemics such as metformin or a sulfonylurea.

Incretin mimetics (e.g. exenatide, liraglutide) improve glycemic control and stabilize blood glucose postprandially by mimicking the actions of glucagon-like peptide (GLP)-1. They also induce significant weight loss. They are currently only available in injectable form, and often cause nausea.

Dipeptidyl peptidase (DPP)-4 inhibitors (e.g. sitagliptin, vildagliptin) have similar effects to incretin mimetics but are weight neutral.

Insulin is recommended when satisfactory control of blood glucose cannot be achieved with oral hypoglycemic therapy.

Bariatric surgery (see Chapter 9) has a high success rate in patients with diabetes. Some studies have reported a postoperative cure rate of 90%, which lasts, particularly if surgery is performed early in the course of the disease.

Polycystic ovary syndrome

PCOS is the most common endocrine disturbance in women: at least 11% of obese women with type 2 diabetes also have PCOS. Diagnostic criteria are given in Table 4.3, and investigations for PCOS in Table 4.4.

PCOS is characterized by androgenic effects, which may include acne, alopecia and hirsutism, typically of male distribution, including chin, upper lip, chest, back, abdomen, upper arms, thighs and buttocks. Ovulation is disordered, and oligomenorrhea or amenorrhea may occur.

Women with PCOS are at increased risk of cardiovascular disease and other related comorbidities, including non-alcoholic fatty liver disease, obstructive sleep apnea (OSA) and certain cancers.

TABLE 4.3

Diagnosis of polycystic ovary syndrome

Two of the following three criteria should be present:

- oligo- or anovulation
- clinical or biochemical evidence of hyperandrogenism
- polycystic ovaries*

*An ovary with ≥ 12 follicles measuring 2–9 mm in diameter, and/or increased ovarian volume (> 10 cm^3)

TABLE 4.4

Tests for polycystic ovary syndrome

	Normal range (may vary with local laboratory assays)	Comments
Pelvic ultrasound	To assess ovarian morphology and endometrial thickness	Transabdominal scan adequate in women who are not sexually active
Testosterone	0.5–3.5 nmol/L	Measurement of other androgens unnecessary unless total testosterone > 5 nmol/L, in which case referral is indicated
Sex hormone binding globulin (SHBG)	16–119 nmol/L	
Free androgen index: (testosterone / SHBG) × 100	< 5	Insulin suppresses SHBG, resulting in a high free androgen index in the presence of normal total testosterone level
Luteinizing hormone (LH) Follicle-stimulating hormone (FSH)	2–10 IU/L 2–8 IU/L	FSH and LH are best measured during days 1–3 of menstrual bleed Take random samples if oligo-/ amenorrhea
Prolactin Thyroid-stimulating hormone	< 500 mU/L 0.5–5 IU/L	Measure in case of oligo-/ amenorrhea
Insulin resistance		Measured by glucose tolerance test; fasting insulin not measured routinely

Treatment. As insulin resistance is the main precursor to PCOS, the mainstays of treatment are dietary modification and increased physical activity, as described above and in Chapters 6 and 7. Insulin sensitizers, particularly metformin, have an important role; they may improve hyperandrogenism and can restore fertility. (Metformin is unlicensed in PCOS.)

A combined oral contraceptive may be prescribed to regulate the menstrual cycle and protect the endometrium by the induction of regular withdrawal bleeds. Ovulation and fertility can be induced in secondary care by anti-estrogens such as clomifene (clomiphene), although ultrasound monitoring is essential because of the risk of multiple pregnancy.

Hirsutism often improves with weight loss and increased physical activity together with the use of a combined oral contraceptive, which increases levels of sex hormone binding globulin (SHBG) and lowers free androgen levels. Androgen receptor antagonists such as aldactone, where available, may be useful. Cosmetic therapies include electrolysis, waxing, bleaching and lasers. Eflornithine, which inhibits the enzyme ornithine decarboxylase in hair follicles, has been developed as a topical treatment.

Atherogenic dyslipidemia

Atherogenic dyslipidemia, also known as the 'lipid triad', refers to the specific lipid changes associated with insulin resistance and the metabolic syndrome:

- moderately raised triglycerides
- an increased preponderance of small dense LDL particles
- low levels of HDL cholesterol.

'The hypertriglyceridemic waist' has been proposed as the easiest way to identify high-risk patients in the clinic. The combination of abdominal obesity with raised plasma triglycerides identifies an individual at high risk for cardiovascular disease (Figure 4.4). Waist circumference and weight gain are the strongest predictors of early atherosclerosis in apparently healthy adults.

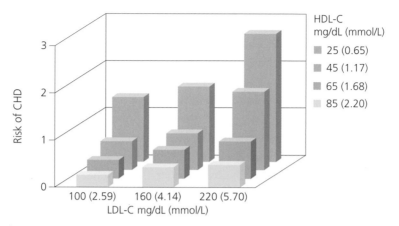

Figure 4.4 High-density lipoprotein cholesterol (HDL-C) as an independent predictor of coronary heart disease (CHD). LDL-C, low-density lipoprotein cholesterol. Reprinted from Gordon T et al. *Am J Med* 1977;62:707–14 with permission from Elsevier.

Epidemiology. Dyslipidemia develops progressively as BMI increases from 21 kg/m², increasing the risk of CHD by a factor of 3.6. It is estimated that about 38% of patients with BMI above 27 kg/m² have hypercholesterolemia. The Framingham study revealed that cholesterol increased by 12 mg/dL (0.3 mmol/L) for every 10% gain in weight. Up to 80% of patients with a waist measurement of at least 90 cm and a plasma triglyceride concentration above 2 mmol/L (0.02 mg/dL) possess the atherogenic combination of lipids that increases the risk of CHD by a factor of 20.

Measurement of apolipoproteins. While the ratio of total cholesterol to HDL cholesterol expresses the overall risk of disease from dyslipidemia, it is now accepted that the ratio of apolipoprotein (apo)B (the primary protein constituent of LDL) to apoA1 (one of the major apolipoproteins in HDL) is a more precise measurement of atherogenic risk: a large number of small apoB particles is more atherogenic than a small number of large apoA1 particles. The number of particles can be assessed accurately in clinical trials by measuring apoB, as there is one molecule of apoB per LDL particle; a high apoB:apoA1 ratio expresses a high risk for CHD.

Management

Weight loss significantly improves the lipid profile. Extensive Cochrane analyses have reported that a weight loss of 10 kg will induce a reduction in total cholesterol of about 0.25 mmol/L (9.75 mg/dL; approximately 5%). The American National Cholesterol Education Program reported that every 3 kg of diet-induced weight loss was accompanied by an increase in HDL cholesterol of 0.025 nmol/L (1 mg/dL), and it is widely accepted that 10% weight loss will induce a reduction in LDL cholesterol of approximately 15% and an increase in HDL of 8%, with a 10% fall in total cholesterol.

Figure 4.5 demonstrates improvement in lipid profile with weight loss, based on a meta-analysis of 70 studies. During weight loss, HDL levels decrease initially but then increase once weight loss has stabilized. Otherwise the greatest improvements in serum lipid concentrations tend to occur in the first 4–8 weeks of weight loss.

Dietary management. The effects of dietary changes are probably due partly to weight loss per se and partly to the effects of a more appropriate diet. The Finnish North Karelia study showed that a

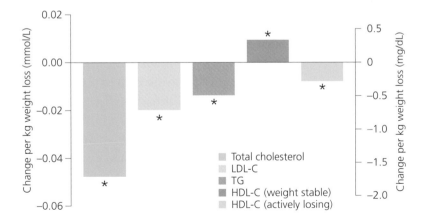

Figure 4.5 Results of a meta-analysis of 70 trials, showing that weight loss improves plasma lipids. Reproduced with permission from Dattilo and Kris-Etherton 1992. HDL-C, high-density lipoprotein cholesterol; LDL-C, low-density lipoprotein cholesterol; TG, triglycerides. *$p \leq 0.05$.

trebling in vegetable consumption over a 15-year period was accompanied by a substantial reduction in saturated fat intake, a substantial decline in salt intake and a 15% decrease in total serum cholesterol concentrations. Remarkably, however, these changes induced an increase, rather than a decrease, in the average BMI of the population, highlighting the importance of optimal nutrition in improving health.

Anti-obesity drug therapy in conjunction with lifestyle changes has been shown to improve lipid profiles in obese patients. Various studies have shown that orlistat reduces total and LDL cholesterol to a greater extent than weight loss alone. Sibutramine appears to have some benefit in increasing HDL cholesterol levels.

Inflammation

Obesity, particularly severe obesity, or the presence of obesity-related comorbidities such as diabetes and cardiovascular disease are associated with increased plasma levels of inflammatory cytokines and activation of the acute phase response, as reflected by levels of C-reactive protein. Although adipocytes themselves secrete pro-inflammatory cytokines, they are predominantly produced by activated macrophages present in adipose tissue, particularly when it accumulates viscerally. A number of the cardiometabolic complications of obesity are likely to be caused, or at the very least exacerbated, by this pro-inflammatory state. In contrast, plasma levels of adiponectin, a cytokine derived from adipocytes that is associated with an antidiabetogenic effect, are lower in obese patients with insulin resistance. Levels decrease further as the metabolic state deteriorates and type 2 diabetes mellitus develops.

A diet high in saturated fat, the presence of OSA and psychosocial stress all aggravate the pro-inflammatory state.

The prothrombotic state

The prothrombotic state linked with obesity and the metabolic syndrome refers to changes in coagulation factors that promote increased blood viscosity and hypercoagulability, arterial thrombosis and inflammation, and increasing plaque and thrombus formation in the arterial wall. The prothrombotic state is characterized by endothelial dysfunction, enhanced LDL oxidation, promotion of platelet aggregation, activation of factor VII, and increases in factors IX and X, prothrombin and plasminogen activation inhibitor-1. Peroxisome proliferator-activated receptor-α may also play a role in atherogenic dyslipidemia and inflammation.

Hypertension

Obesity is a risk factor for the development of hypertension. Blood pressure should therefore be measured as part of the screening process once an individual is identified as being overweight. It should be measured with a sufficiently large cuff designed for obese individuals (otherwise the reading will be abnormally high), which should be readily accessible in order to avoid embarrassment to patient and physician.

Epidemiology. More than 85% of patients with hypertension have a BMI of 25 kg/m^2 or more. The risk of hypertension is increased fivefold among obese people compared with their lean counterparts, and in up to two-thirds blood pressure is raised as a direct consequence of excess weight. Individuals who are 20% overweight have an eightfold chance of developing hypertension. The Framingham study showed that each 4.5 kg weight gain led to an increase in systolic blood pressure of about 4.3 mmHg; 15% gain in weight was associated with an 18% increase in systolic blood pressure.

The Physicians' Health Study, which observed 13 500 normotensive men, discovered that 4920 participants developed hypertension after a median 14.5 years. Higher baseline BMI, even within the 'normal' range, was consistently associated with increased risk of hypertension. The Asia-Pacific Cohort Collaboration Study, which involved 26–33 cohorts of more than 300 000 adults followed up for almost 7 years, showed that each unit change in BMI was associated with a 9% difference in ischemic heart disease events, and a change of about 8% in hypertension-related deaths and ischemic strokes.

A recent study of 20 000 male and a similar number of female high-school students revealed hemodynamic abnormalities – hypertension and raised heart rate – in obese adolescents. Increases in both systolic and diastolic blood pressure were associated with high resting heart rate, and this observed clustering increased with the degree of obesity, probably explained by impaired autonomic nerve function.

It is clear from studies such as these that screening of obese individuals for possible covert hypertension should be a priority, and will identify a large number of high-risk individuals whose risk can be successfully modified, and death prevented, by appropriate lifestyle changes and drug treatment.

Mechanism of obesity-related hypertension. Increased renal sodium reabsorption and blood volume expansion are central features in the development of obesity-related hypertension. Hyperinsulinemia leads to renal salt retention. Overweight is also associated with increased sympathetic activity, an effect that may be mediated by leptin, a protein expressed in and secreted by adipocytes. The renin–angiotensin–aldosterone system has also been causally implicated in obesity-related hypertension, partly because of activation by increased sympathetic activity, and perhaps also because angiotensinogen is expressed in and secreted by adipose tissue. Low levels of the adipocyte-derived cytokine adiponectin, high circulating levels of free fatty acids and increased vascular production of endothelin-1 have also been implicated in mediating the effect of obesity to increase blood pressure.

Dietary factors are also important: excess intake of saturated fats and refined carbohydrates increase systolic and diastolic blood pressure. Salt intake is more likely to be associated with hypertension in obesity.

Management

Weight loss through dietary modification and increased physical activity is the cornerstone of the treatment and prevention of both obesity and hypertension, whether they occur alone or together. Caloric restriction, reduced intake of refined carbohydrate and saturated fat, very low salt intake and increased fiber intake (from whole grains, salads, vegetables and fruit) are beneficial, regardless of weight. Reductions of 1 mmHg in systolic pressure and 2 mmHg in diastolic pressure for each 1% reduction in weight have been reported.

Pharmacotherapy. Angiotensin-converting enzyme (ACE) inhibitors, angiotensin receptor blockers (ARBs) and calcium channel blockers can be used in conjunction with weight loss for the treatment of high blood pressure in obese individuals. Both ACE inhibitors and ARBs have been associated with favorable metabolic properties and end-organ protection in addition to their antihypertensive effects. Beta-blockers should be avoided because of the risk of weight gain.

Key points – cardiometabolic consequences

- Obesity is important because of its effect on cardiometabolic status and risk.
- The metabolic syndrome defines the clustering of cardiovascular risk factors under the umbrella of obesity.
- Type 2 diabetes is the comorbidity most closely linked with obesity.
- Lipid disorders and hypertension are exacerbated by obesity and add to cardiovascular risk.
- Weight loss rapidly and effectively reduces cardiovascular risk and improves glycemic control.

Key references

Avenell A, Broom J, Brown TJ et al. Systematic review of the long-term effects and economic consequences of treatments for obesity and implications for health improvement. *Health Technol Assess* 2004;8:iii–iv,1–182.

Baba R, Koketsu M, Nagashima M et al. Adolescent obesity adversely affects blood pressure and resting heart rate. *Circ J* 2007;71:722–6.

Chrostowska M, Szczech R, Narkiewicz K. Antihypertensive therapy in the obese hypertensive patient. *Curr Opin Nephrol Hypertens* 2006;15:487–92.

Dattilo AM, Kris-Etherton PM. Effects of weight reduction on blood lipids and lipoproteins: a meta-analysis. *Am J Clin Nutr* 1992;56:320–8

Ford ES, Giles WH, Dietz WH. Prevalence of the metabolic syndrome among US adults: findings from the third National Health and Nutrition Examination Survey. *JAMA* 2002;287:356–9.

Gelber RP, Gaziano JM, Manson JE et al. A prospective study of body mass index and the risk of developing hypertension in men. *Am J Hypertens* 2007;20:370–7.

Haslam D, James WP. Obesity. *Lancet* 2005;366:1197–209.

MacGregor GA, Kaplan NM. *Fast Facts: Hypertension*, 3rd edn. Oxford: Health Press, 2006.

Moghetti P, Castello R, Negri C et al. Metformin effects on clinical features, endocrine and metabolic profiles, and insulin sensitivity in polycystic ovary syndrome: a randomized, double-blind, placebo-controlled 6-month trial, followed by open, long-term clinical evaluation. *J Clin Endocrinol Metab* 2000;85: 139–46.

Pietinen P, Lahti-Koski M, Vartiainen E, Puska P. Nutrition and cardiovascular disease in Finland since the early 1970s: a success story. *J Nutr Health Aging* 2001;5:150–4.

Sacks FM, Svetkey LP, Vollmer WM et al. Effects on blood pressure of reduced dietary sodium and the Dietary Approaches to Stop Hypertension (DASH) diet. DASH-Sodium Collaborative Research Group. *N Engl J Med* 2001;344:3–10.

Scobie IN, Samaras K. *Fast Facts: Diabetes Mellitus*, 3rd edn. Oxford: Health Press, 2009.

Sniderman A, Durrington P. *Fast Facts: Hyperlipidemia*, 4th edn. Oxford: Health Press, 2008.

Wadden TA, Anderson DA, Foster GD. Two-year changes in lipids and lipoproteins associated with the maintenance of a 5% to 10% reduction in initial weight: some findings and some questions. *Obes Res* 1999;7:170–8.

5   Other consequences

Respiratory disorders

The major respiratory complications of obesity are shown in Table 5.1, all of which impair quality of life. Patients with obesity also commonly develop hypoventilation and sleep apnea syndromes, with attenuated hypoxic and hypercapnic ventilatory responsiveness. The final result is hypoxemia, pulmonary hypertension and progressively worsening disability.

Lung function. Conventional respiratory function tests are only mildly affected by obesity except in extreme cases. However, obesity is associated with decreased functional residual capacity (FRC) and expiratory reserve volume, a high closing-volume-to-FRC ratio, associated with closure of peripheral lung units, abnormalities of the ventilation-to-perfusion ratio and hypoxemia, especially in the supine position. Obesity is associated with reduced lung volume, which is linked with airway narrowing. However, in men, airway narrowing is greater than that due to reduced lung volume alone. In children, severe obesity is associated with reductions in basal forced vital capacity, forced expiratory volume in 1 second and peak expiratory flow, and increased airway responsiveness.

TABLE 5.1

Major respiratory complications of obesity

- Heightened demand for ventilation
- Diminished respiratory compliance
- Increased work of breathing
- Inefficiency of respiratory muscles
- Increased dyspnea
- Decreased exercise capacity

Obstructive sleep apnea (OSA). Although obesity is a major risk factor for OSA, this condition aggregates in families, a relationship that is not simply explained by obesity. For children, obesity at the time of diagnosis is a major risk for OSA persisting after treatment, regardless of the severity of initial disease.

Obesity hypoventilation syndrome is defined as a combination of obesity and chronic hypoventilation; it ultimately results in pulmonary hypertension, cor pulmonale and probable early death.

Asthma. The extent to which obesity contributes to asthma and airway hyperresponsiveness is uncertain. Central obesity is associated with an increased risk of non-atopic asthma. Obese patients with asthma are less likely than non-obese patients to achieve optimal control of their disease.

Management. Weight reduction and physical activity reverse the respiratory complications of obesity.

Liver and gastrointestinal disorders

Non-alcoholic fatty liver disease (NAFLD). The spectrum of NAFLD ranges from simple steatosis (fat deposition), which has a benign prognosis, to non-alcoholic steatohepatitis (NASH), which is associated with inflammation as a consequence of fat deposition and cirrhosis. Hepatic steatosis is the primary abnormality in patients with NAFLD and is associated with excess visceral adipose tissue, insulin resistance and hypertriglyceridemia. Activation of multiple pro-inflammatory cytokines results in NASH.

NASH due to NAFLD is becoming a new major health problem as a result of rising levels of obesity. Hepatic steatosis has an adverse influence on the progression of other liver diseases, including chronic hepatitis C virus infection and alcoholic liver disease. The presence of hepatic steatosis in patients with type 2 diabetes does not appear to affect apolipoprotein (apo)B levels, but potentially increases atherogenesis by increasing triglycerides, reducing HDL levels and increasing small dense LDL (see page 49). NAFLD may be both a marker and an early mediator of atherosclerosis

Raised alanine aminotransferase (ALT) activity may indicate the presence of NAFLD, although it lacks sensitivity and underestimates the true prevalence.

With the rising prevalence of obesity, fatty liver has become the most common liver abnormality in children and adolescents aged 2–19 years; some degree of excess liver fat occurs in approximately 10% of children, although severe NASH is uncommon.

Management involves weight loss and aggressive control of risk factors. Weight reduction and increased physical activity should be priorities in obese patients to improve insulin sensitivity. Orlistat improves serum ALT levels and steatosis on ultrasound in patients with NAFLD. Bariatric surgery (see Chapter 9) reduces the fat, inflammation, and even the fibrosis, in well-documented NASH.

Gastroesophageal reflux disease (GERD). Obesity is associated with an increase in symptomatic GERD and hospitalization for GERD-related complications. In addition to the effect of baseline bodyweight, an increase in bodyweight of more than 4 kg (10 lb) is associated with new onset of reflux symptoms. The condition invariably resolves with weight loss or at least is substantially ameliorated.

Lower gastrointestinal tract disorders. The relationship between obesity and abdominal pain and diarrhea may be related to poor nutrition (high fat, inadequate fruit/fiber intake) and limited physical activity. The regularity of physical activity may be the major predictive factor.

Although the etiologic relationship between obesity and diverticular complications remains unclear, patients with perforations and recurrent diverticulitis are significantly more obese than those who remain asymptomatic or have one episode.

Lower gastrointestinal function is improved by a diet that is low in saturated fat and based on unprocessed foods and abundant natural fiber, together with water for hydration rather than soft drinks or fruit juice, and regular physical activity.

Gallbladder disease. Obese patients are at increased risk for biliary disease, with a higher incidence of cholelithiasis, cholecystitis and cholesterolosis.

The incidence of gallbladder disease is increasing in children and adolescents concomitant with the increasing incidence of obesity.

Weight loss does not benefit patients with biliary disease, and cholecystectomy is usually required. Rapid weight loss may precipitate acute cholelithiasis.

Reproductive consequences

Table 5.2 lists the reproductive consequences of obesity.

Men

Plasma testosterone. Obesity, particularly when visceral and accompanied by impairment of glucose metabolism, is associated with low plasma total testosterone, but not free testosterone levels, as a result of a decrease in sex hormone binding globulin (SHBG); obesity and metabolic syndrome leads to low testosterone levels rather than vice versa. OSA associated with obesity decreases both total and free testosterone.

Total testosterone should not be measured in isolation in obese men. The SHBG should be determined and free testosterone calculated. A low testosterone level should prompt screening for the metabolic complications of obesity and OSA.

Weight loss, reversal of the metabolic abnormalities and treatment of OSA will improve plasma testosterone.

TABLE 5.2

Reproductive consequences of obesity

Male	Female
Low plasma testosterone	Urinary incontinence
Erectile dysfunction	Infertility
Lower urinary tract symptoms	Polycystic ovary syndrome (see pages 47–9)
Poor semen quality	Complications in pregnancy
Low sperm count	Breast cancer
Reduced fertility	Endometrial cancer

Erectile dysfunction is a marker of cardiovascular risk and is associated with visceral obesity primarily as a result of associated metabolic abnormalities that induce endothelial dysfunction. Weight loss through a lifestyle modification program is associated with improvements in erectile dysfunction in obese men.

Lower urinary tract symptoms (LUTS). There are also relationships between visceral obesity, components of the metabolic syndrome, OSA and LUTS, particularly nocturia. Weight gain and central adiposity in adulthood are particularly associated with an increased risk of LUTS.

There is a close relationship between LUTS, erectile dysfunction and the metabolic syndrome; LUTS responds well to weight loss.

Semen quality and fertility. Obese men may have fewer sertoli cells than men of normal weight. Semen quality, sperm count and fertility are all compromised by overweight and obesity. The effect of weight loss on these abnormalities remains unclear.

Women

Urinary incontinence. The presence and severity of urinary incontinence in women are associated with increasing BMI or waist circumference. A large waist circumference may be associated with stress incontinence whereas high BMI is associated with urge and mixed, but not stress, urinary incontinence. Urinary incontinence also has an adverse effect on sexual function in obese women.

Infertility. Even in the absence of polycystic ovary syndrome (PCOS), obesity contributes to anovulation, menstrual irregularities, reduced rates of conception and response to fertility treatment.

Treatment of obesity by a combination of healthy nutrition and regular physical activity may restore fertility and responsiveness to assisted reproduction and should always be the initial approach. Weight loss following bariatric surgery often restores fertility, and pregnancy is feasible and usually successful.

Complications of pregnancy and childbirth. Pregnancy in obese women is more likely to be complicated by hypertensive conditions, pre-eclampsia, gestational diabetes, infection and thromboembolic events. Induction of labor is more likely to be required and there is an increased risk of cesarean section, which in itself is associated with greater risk in obese women. Premature birth, stillbirth and perinatal death are more likely in women who are overweight or obese, and the newborns are more likely to be macrosomic, to require treatment for jaundice or hypoglycemia or to have a congenital anomaly. Pregnancy is discussed in more detail in Chapter 10.

Cancer

Large prospective studies show significant associations between obesity and several cancers, including cancers of the prostate, female breast, colon, endometrium, kidney, esophagus and liver (hepatocellular carcinoma).

Survival is decreased in obese women with cancer; this may be disease specific, the result of comorbid illnesses or a reflection of response to treatment. Obesity also increases the risk of complications from surgery and radiation therapy. There is no current consensus regarding appropriate dosing of chemotherapy in the obese patient.

Prostate cancer. Obesity may impact on the risk, detection and outcome of prostate cancer. While BMI has been shown to be inversely related to prostate cancer risk, prostate cancer in obese men is characterized by worse pathological features and higher biochemical relapse rates. Obesity does not affect the utility of prostate-specific antigen as a marker of prostate cancer.

Breast cancer. The relationship between obesity and breast cancer risk as well as the clinical behavior of the disease is complicated. In postmenopausal women, particularly the elderly, obesity is positively associated with risk for breast cancer, whereas before menopause increased bodyweight is inversely related to breast cancer risk. The mechanisms by which bodyweight and obesity affect risk have been related to estrogenic activity in both pre- and postmenopausal breast cancer. Obesity has also been related to advanced disease at diagnosis and with a poor prognosis.

Endometrial cancer. Excess adiposity, weight gain and weight cycling are associated with an increased risk of endometrial cancer; inactivity and high energy intake are major risk factors for endometrial cancer independent of BMI. The presence of hypertension and relative hyperglycemia are significant markers of risk, especially among the heaviest women.

Colorectal cancer. Bodyweight and BMI increase the risk of colon cancer in men, but not in women. This discrepancy may be related to differences in fat distribution between the sexes or the use of hormone replacement therapy (HRT) in women, which lowers the risk of colon cancer. In contrast, waist circumference, a marker of abdominal obesity, is associated with colon cancer risk in men and women, although this too may vary depending on HRT use in postmenopausal women.

Renal cell cancer (RCC) accounts for 2% of all new cancer cases worldwide but incidence is rising steadily. Cigarette smoking and obesity are the most consistently established causal risk factors, accounting for more than 20% and 30% of RCCs, respectively. Obesity increases the risk of RCC among women irrespective of fat distribution, whereas low hip circumference is related to increased risk of RCC in men. Hypertension appears to influence development of RCC, although the mechanism is unknown. As with other cancers, fruit and vegetable consumption appears to have a protective effect.

Gastrointestinal tract cancers. Alcohol, tobacco and obesity interact to increase the risk of hepatocellular carcinoma. Obesity also increases the risk of adenocarcinoma of the lower esophagus and gastric cardia (but not non-cardia gastric adenocarcinoma) and pancreatic cancer, which may be related to intake of refined carbohydrates, glucose intolerance, hyperinsulinemia and physical inactivity.

Disorders of the bones, joints and soft tissues

Obesity is a key risk factor in the onset and progression of musculoskeletal conditions of the hip, knee, ankle, foot and shoulder. In addition to the effect of obesity on bones and joints, emerging evidence indicates that obesity may also have a profound effect on soft tissue structures such as tendons, fascia and cartilage.

Overweight children and adolescents also show greater prevalence of reported fractures, musculoskeletal discomfort, impaired mobility and lower-extremity malalignment than their normal-weight peers, which may be part of the cycle that perpetuates the accumulation of excess weight.

Osteoarthritis is the third leading cause of life-years lost due to disability. Obesity and joint injury are important potentially modifiable risk factors for the development of osteoarthritis. Obesity is also an important predictor of osteoarthritis progression. Overweight at any time is related to knee osteoarthritis. A moderate increase in BMI, even within the normal weight range, is significantly related to knee osteoarthritis among men. Obesity is also strongly related to hip osteoarthritis, back pain and osteoarthritis in other joints, for example thumb carpometacarpal osteoarthritis, in both sexes.

Each pound (454 g) of weight lost results in a fourfold reduction in the load exerted on the knee per step during daily activities. An intensive weight-loss program that involves an energy-deficit diet and exercise training improves physical function in older obese adults with osteoarthritis of the knee. Greatest improvements in function are seen in those with the greatest weight loss. Surgically induced weight loss (see Chapter 9) is an effective, rapid and dependable means of reversing the radiological signs of early changes associated with osteoarthritis.

Joint replacement surgery. Total knee replacement improves mobility, enhancing the success of subsequent weight-loss therapy. However, successful treatment of lower-extremity arthritis may not lead to weight loss, and obesity should be treated as an independent disease that is not necessarily the result of inactivity from arthritis.

Moderate obesity does not appear to affect the outcome of hip or knee replacement surgery in patients with arthritis. Other data suggest that BMI of 30 kg/m^2 and higher has a negative effect on the outcome of total knee replacement; outcomes in those with a BMI greater than 40 kg/m^2 are clearly poorer. Preoperative weight loss and an ongoing weight-maintenance program are therefore advisable.

Obesity does not appear to confer an independent risk for hip or knee revision procedures.

Soft tissues. Obesity increases the risk of plantar fasciitis, achilles tendon rupture, meniscal tears, carpal tunnel syndrome and peripheral edema.

Mobility and disability. Among elderly community dwellers there is a strong association between obesity and disability, including mobility and independent activities of daily living. The risks of musculoskeletal disorders, arthritis, rheumatism and personal care disability are significantly elevated, even in those who are overweight.

Mental health and cognitive function

Community samples of adolescents and adults indicate that depressive symptoms and psychiatric morbidity are not significantly higher in obese than normal-weight groups. However, the prevalence of psychiatric morbidity, most commonly depression, is increased in patients seeking treatment for obesity (40–60%), and extreme obesity is associated with an increased risk for depression.

Obesity in adolescence may be associated with depression in young adulthood. In women, being overweight or obese in both adolescence and adulthood may be a risk for later depression. In men, abdominal obesity may be closely related to concomitant depression.

Stigmatization is a common experience; more frequent exposure to stigmatization increases the psychological distress.

Management. Depression and other psychiatric conditions should be managed before starting a weight-loss program. The selective serotonin-reuptake inhibitors (SSRIs) tend not to lead to weight gain and may be associated with some weight loss (see Table 3.2, page 35).

Lifestyle approaches, particularly those incorporating some form of cognitive behavior therapy, have been shown to induce modest weight loss, improve emotional well-being and reduce distress, improvements that were maintained or continued at 1 year follow-up. Sustained weight loss, such as that achieved by bariatric surgery, can substantially improve self-esteem and quality of life, although this tends to be less in patients with depression before surgery and in those with less weight loss.

In some patients, weight loss of more than 5 kg may exacerbate depression because of the rigid restraint of eating.

Cognitive function. After controlling for age and other possible confounding factors, performance on all cognitive tests is inversely related to BMI. Overweight and obese adults (BMI > 25 kg/m^2) exhibit poorer executive function than normal-weight adults. The diminished performance on tests of motor speed, manual dexterity and executive function (i.e. response inhibition) due to obesity is compounded by increased blood pressure (systolic or diastolic). There are no data on the effect of weight loss on these measures of cognitive function.

Overall quality of life. Morbid obesity contributes to the impairment of all domains of health-related quality of life. Weight loss improves quality of life; the greatest improvements occur in response to weight loss following bariatric surgery.

Neurological problems

Cerebrovascular disease and peripheral neuropathy. Apart from overt diabetes mellitus, it is increasingly recognized that impaired glucose tolerance and metabolic syndrome associated with obesity are risk factors for cerebrovascular events and peripheral neuropathy.

Benign intracranial hypertension is a syndrome characterized by the abnormal elevation of intracranial pressure with normal-composition cerebrospinal fluid in the absence of ventriculomegaly or an intracranial expansive lesion. The syndrome is most frequently seen in women and is strongly associated with obesity and a recent increase in weight. Presenting features include headache, alterations of visual acuity, double vision and nausea with some vomiting. Benign intracranial hypertension is resolved in some patients with morbid obesity by substantial weight loss, such as that induced by bariatric surgery.

Surgery and anesthetic risk

All surgery, but abdominal surgery in particular, is associated with increased morbidity and mortality in the obese. Table 5.3 shows the main complications of surgery in obese patients. Every effort should be made to identify and reduce obesity-related comorbidities, as well as weight (if necessary using a very-low-calorie diet; see Chapter 6), before surgery. It is particularly important to identify and appropriately manage significant OSA. Ask the patient about loud snoring, day-time somnolence, frequent nocturia and morning headaches; if present, obtain a sleep study.

TABLE 5.3

Complications of surgery in obese patients

- Wound infection
- Chest infection
- Respiratory failure
- Deep venous thrombosis
- Pulmonary embolism
- Incisional hernia
- Anesthetic risk from related comorbidities
    - Cardiovascular (hypertension, ischemic heart disease, right heart failure)
    - Respiratory (restrictive, obstructive sleep apnea, central hypoventilation)
    - Gastrointestinal (gastroesophageal reflux disease)
    - Metabolic (diabetes mellitus)
    - Neurological (autonomic neuropathy)

Key points – other consequences

- Obesity is associated with potentially serious physical and psychological consequences and almost every system in the body may be affected.
- The distribution of excess body fat determines the nature of the adverse consequences of obesity.
- Obese patients should be assessed for obesity-related comorbidities.
- Consider and manage obesity in all patients presenting with problems that may be related to obesity, or where obesity may confer a risk (surgery, pregnancy).
- The metabolic consequences of excess weight may respond to as little as 5–10% weight loss; much greater weight loss is required for other comorbidities (e.g. obstructive sleep apnea).

Key references

Frey C, Zamora J. The effects of obesity on orthopaedic foot and ankle pathology. *Foot Ankle Int* 2007;28:996–9.

García Hidalgo L. Dermatological complications of obesity. *Am J Clin Dermatol* 2002;3:497–506.

Hampel H, Abraham NS, El-Serag HB. Meta-analysis: obesity and the risk for gastroesophageal reflux disease and its complications. *Ann Intern Med* 2005;143:199–211.

Jubber AS. Respiratory complications of obesity. *Int J Clin Pract* 2004;58:573–80.

Larsen SH, Wagner G, Heitmann BL. Sexual function and obesity. *Int J Obes* 2007;31:1189–98.

Mah PM, Wittert GA. Obesity and testicular function. *Mol Cell Endocrinol* 2009 Jun 18 [Epub ahead of print].

Malnick SD, Knobler H. The medical complications of obesity. *QJM* 2006;99:565–79.

Pischon T, Nöthlings U, Boeing H. Obesity and cancer. *Proc Nutr Soc* 2008;67:128–45.

Satpathy HK, Fleming A, Frey D et al. Maternal obesity and pregnancy. *Postgrad Med* 2008; 120:E01–9.

Talen MR, Mann MM. Obesity and mental health. *Prim Care* 2009;36: 287–305.

Energy balance

Food is metabolized and converted to energy, which is used in the following three ways:

- basal metabolic rate (BMR) – the energy used to keep the bodily functions ticking over accounts for 60–70% of energy expenditure; apart from genetic factors, variability in BMR depends on lean body mass, in particular skeletal muscle, and the activity of the sympathetic nervous system
- thermogenesis – energy used to process and digest the foods that provide energy, normally around 10%
- physical activity – energy used in performing muscular activity, including daily tasks and scheduled exercise; accounts for 15–30% of daily energy expenditure.

Energy that is in excess of requirements is stored as fat. A negative energy balance, regardless of how it is achieved, will result in a reduction in fat mass. As proof of this principle, it was recently shown that a specified negative energy balance results in comparable magnitudes of weight loss whether it is achieved entirely by caloric restriction or by a combination of caloric restriction and physical activity. Most people, however, achieve a negative energy balance more easily by reducing their caloric intake than by increased physical activity. For example, a 300 kcal reduction in energy can be achieved by eliminating a small packet of potato chips (crisps), or by substituting two diet sodas for two regular sodas; the alternative is to run 5 km (3 miles) or cycle 8 km in 30 minutes.

A caloric deficit of 500–1000 kcal/day will promote a weight loss of 0.5–1 kg per week. The easiest way to reduce energy intake is to reduce the energy density of the diet. A reduction in bodyweight through caloric restriction will result in a lower daily energy expenditure because of lower BMR and a lower energy cost associated with moving a smaller body mass. Maintenance of weight loss is therefore critically dependent on physical activity.

Dietary approaches to weight management

A number of dietary approaches, based on various macronutrient patterns, are commonly used to achieve weight loss. Most of these popular diets have been found to modestly reduce bodyweight and several cardiac risk factors at 1 year. Dietary adherence is more important than the specific dietary pattern, and overall adherence to any of the diets has been found to be low. It is therefore reasonable to work within the parameters that accommodate the characteristics of a particular patient – culture, lifestyle, understanding, sex, age etc.

Important factors in promoting dietary adherence include convenience, choice and an ongoing behavioral support program. Dietary patterns are described briefly here. Table 6.1 shows the recommended approach. The best diet is based on optimal nutrient composition and the highest likelihood of adherence. Healthy diets focus on fruit and vegetables, whole grains and lean unprocessed meat, chicken and seafood. Up to 30% of energy may come from fat. Intake of saturated (animal) fat should be very limited. The fats consumed should be predominantly of plant origin, for example monounsaturated fatty acids (MUFA; from olive oil) and long-chain polyunsaturated fatty acids (PUFA). A high intake of omega-3 fatty acids (long-chain PUFA mainly from seafood), particularly when intake of saturated fatty

TABLE 6.1

Key strategies for the dietary management of weight loss

- Overall nutritional quality and balance (fresh foods) is key
- Low energy density
- Low fat (< 30%), marked restriction of saturated and trans fatty acids; emphasis on monounsaturated fats and long-chain polyunsaturated fatty acids, in particular omega-3 fatty acids
- Increased fiber, use complex carbohydrates
- Small portion size
- Choice
- Convenience
- Ongoing behavioral strategy required

acids is low, may be associated with lower rates of diabetes, heart disease and less inflammation. Low-fat dairy products are part of a healthy balanced diet. Water rather than fruit juice or soft drinks is the optimum fluid for hydration.

It is the overall quality of the diet that appears to offer protection against 'lifestyle' disease such as metabolic syndrome.

Energy-dense vs nutrient-dense foods. Energy density is defined as the energy (kilocalories) provided by a certain weight (grams) of food. In general, most energy-dense foods are high-fat foods (often dry foods), whereas most foods that contain a lot of water (e.g. fruits, vegetables, soups) have a low energy density. After oxidation, fat generates 9 kcal/g, while carbohydrate and protein generate 4 kcal/g.

Food intake is regulated in part by food weight; since energy-dense foods weigh less for a given amount of energy, more is consumed before the individual feels sated.

Nutrient dense foods provide substantial amounts of vitamins and minerals and relatively fewer calories in a given weight of food. A useful concept is to consider foods in terms of the ratio between nutrient density and energy density. For healthy long-term weight loss and weight maintenance, the food selected should have a high-nutrient but low-energy density.

Standard calorie-restricted diet. High-fat foods are relatively less satiating than iso-energetic portions of high-protein foods or carbohydrate-containing foods with a high fiber content. Many epidemiological studies have shown that a relatively high intake of dietary fat, in particular saturated (animal) fat, corresponds with increased obesity. Reducing intake of saturated fat and refined carbohydrates facilitates weight loss and forms the basis of the most standard dietary approach. Approximately 30% of calories should come from fat. Saturated fat should comprise less than 7% of total calories. Complex carbohydrates from vegetables, fruits and whole grains should be the main source of carbohydrate, enabling a daily fiber intake of 20–30 g.

Despite the widespread promotion of these guidelines, however, the incidence of obesity has continued to rise. Recent data suggest that the problem relates not so much to the guidelines themselves but to:
- failure to adhere to the guidelines
- misguided consumption of highly processed carbohydrate-rich, energy-dense foods that are marketed as 'low fat'
- inadequate intake of fiber from fruit and vegetables
- consumption of sugared drinks
- snacking.

Ultimately, caloric restriction remains the most important factor, as evidenced by data from a recent meta-analysis of randomized clinical trials that compared diets of different macronutrient composition and found no difference in weight loss between diet groups.

Epidemiological data have linked sugar-sweetened beverages to adult and childhood obesity. At both a population and individual level, a reduction in sugar-sweetened beverages (including fruit juice and flavored milks) may be the best single prescription to reduce caloric intake without compromising the intake of essential nutrients.

Manipulation of macronutrients

Fatty acids. There is a relationship between intake of trans and saturated fatty acids and cardiovascular risk. A healthy diet ideally contains no trans fatty acids. Saturated fatty acids impair endothelial function, increase cardiovascular risk, impair glucose tolerance and increase the risk of type 2 diabetes.

Long-chain polyunsaturated fats, and particularly omega-3 fatty acids (long-chain n-3 PUFA), have the combined benefits of lowering triglyceride levels and raising HDL, as well as having favorable effects on insulin resistance and inflammation. They also reduce cardiovascular events in high-risk patients. Incorporation of long-chain n-3 PUFA has been shown to improve risk factors associated with cardiovascular disease when incorporated into a weight-loss program.

Calcium. Diets that are high in calcium, particularly of dairy origin, are associated with lower bodyweights in population studies and may prevent excess weight gain. A healthy diet contains liberal amounts of low-fat milk, natural yogurt and cottage cheese.

Fiber. The epidemiological evidence showing that dietary fiber prevents obesity is strong. BMI, bodyweight and body fat are all inversely related to fiber intake at all levels of fat intake after adjusting for confounding factors. An increase in dietary fiber may assist in weight control and reduce cardiometabolic risk by increasing satiety and therefore decreasing food intake and fat mass, improving glucose metabolism, insulinemia and the blood lipid profile, and reducing blood pressure.

The efficacy of dietary fiber differs according to the dietary source (e.g. fruits, legumes or cereals) and the specific chemical structure of the fiber, responsible for its physical properties (i.e. gel-forming capacity) or fermentation capacity in the lower part of the gut. The fermentability of dietary fiber appears to generate specific effects on satiety and glycemia through the release of gut peptides such as glucagon-like peptide (GLP)-1.

Diets that promote weight loss

Any change in the pattern of eating that is associated with a reduction in energy intake will result in weight loss. However, it is important to recognize that the association between an appropriate diet and overall good health goes beyond issues to do with weight control. From a practical standpoint, it is therefore important to determine for any particular patient where energy intake can be reduced and the nutritional quality of the diet improved without causing a significant disruption to lifestyle.

Low-fat, modified-carbohydrate diets. The concept of glycemic index (GI) was developed as a physiological approach to classifying carbohydrates. The GI is defined as the area under the 2-hour postprandial blood glucose concentration curve per 50 g available carbohydrate consumed from a test food, relative to a reference food (either white bread or pure glucose). Glycemic load (GL) is a related concept, and is the product of the GI of the food or beverage portion and the amount of available (i.e. fiber-free) carbohydrate. Low-GI or low-GL diets have some benefit in the management and prevention of diabetes and cardiovascular disease, but in the context of obesity the data are less clear.

A typical Western high-carbohydrate diet based on high-GI foods such as potatoes, breads and low-fat cereal products is digested and absorbed rapidly, resulting in a high GL and increased demand for insulin secretion. In contrast, low-GI foods such as whole grains and pulses benefit weight control by promoting satiety and fat oxidation at the expense of carbohydrate oxidation.

In practice it is difficult to tease out the separate effects of GI, palatability, volume, fiber and other factors that influence satiety responses to realistic meals. Accordingly, when recommending a low-fat diet it is important to ensure that the carbohydrate consumed is appropriate, and that highly processed foods and those with a low fiber content are avoided. Patients should understand that many foods promoted as 'low fat' are high in carbohydrate and low in fiber, and are therefore best avoided. It is important that patients learn to read and interpret food labels, and that food is labeled in the most informative, easy-to-read and impactful manner.

Increased intake of protein relative to carbohydrate. Clinical studies using ad-libitum intake of diets with an increased ratio of protein to carbohydrate ratio have shown relatively greater loss of fat mass, relative preservation of fat-free mass, improved metabolic profile and better weight maintenance.

Mechanisms by which this may occur include:
- increased satiety
- increased thermogenesis
- sparing of lean body mass.

Examples of diets based on these principles include the Zone, South Beach and the Commonwealth Scientific and Industrial Research Organization (CSIRO) Total Wellbeing diets. In these diets, energy intake is derived from approximately:
- 30% protein
- 40% carbohydrate
- 30% fat.

It is important to emphasize that these diets are most effective when the carbohydrates consumed are unprocessed, nutrient-rich and of low energy density. The metabolic benefits of this dietary approach include lower plasma triglyceride levels and reduced postprandial blood glucose levels.

Very-low-fat, high-carbohydrate diet. This type of diet contributes less than 10% kcal per day as fat, is high in carbohydrate and has a moderate protein content. Examples include the Ornish and Pritikin diets advocated by the American Heart Association (AHA) in the 1980s. The Ornish diet is based on plant-based vegetarian foods that are low in fat and high in complex carbohydrates and fiber; less than 10% of the energy intake should be from fat. The Pritikin diet is similarly low in fat (5–10% of energy), cholesterol, protein (10–15%) and highly refined carbohydrates but is high in complex carbohydrates (80%).

Besides weight loss, these diets have the greatest effect in decreasing serum cholesterol concentrations and thus the risk for heart disease. However, low- and very-low-fat diets (< 20% of daily caloric intake from fat) are not that palatable and adherence in the long term is likely to be poor.

High-fat, low-carbohydrate diet. This type of diet, for example the widely publicized (and studied) Atkins diet, characteristically contains less than 20–30 g of carbohydrate per day, has a high fat content (55–65%) and a relatively high protein content. The diet promotes the consumption of high-fat foods and avoidance of vegetables, fruits, breads, cereals, starchy vegetables and most dairy products; a small amount of salad is generally permitted. A variant, Protein Power, focuses more on protein than fat and permits limited intake of fruit and vegetables.

These diets gained public acceptance because of the rapid weight loss and decreased hunger. The initial rapid weight loss is mostly caused by a diuresis due to depletion of glycogen stores in the liver and muscle, coupled with a lower caloric intake because of limited food choices. Although this dietary pattern leads to greater short-term weight loss than other diets, there is no particular weight loss benefit after 12 months, although, like other low-carbohydrate diets, it produces a greater decrease in triglycerides and increase in HDL cholesterol than low-fat diets. These diets are low in fiber, micronutrients and minerals, and high in saturated fat and protein, and a significant increase in LDL cholesterol occurs in some individuals.

This dietary pattern may be a reasonable option for short-term use in 'healthy' ('metabolically fit') obese individuals with appropriate supplementation of fiber, vitamins and minerals, particularly if it seems that this is the only dietary pattern that will promote adherence. The safety of these diets for people with ischemic heart disease, diabetes or kidney disease remains unclear, and there are no long-term outcome data.

Very-low-calorie diets and meal replacements. The term very-low-calorie diet (VLCD) refers to the use of a manufactured meal replacement that provides calories well below the average daily energy expenditure (450–600 Kcals) while at the same time supplying all the essential amino acids, fatty acids, vitamins, minerals and trace elements. An extra 2–2.5 liters of low-calorie or calorie-free fluid is required. Fiber should be added, since constipation is likely to occur. One sachet of a commercially available fiber preparation (e.g. Benefiber) can be added to each sachet of meal replacement.

VLCDs should form part of a comprehensive overall management program that includes behavioral management (see Chapter 8) and an ongoing lifestyle management program, as short-term approaches to reducing obesity are inevitably followed by regain of all of the weight lost. VLCDs should only be used in appropriate circumstances and after careful assessment. Where appropriate, they may be used in conjunction with appropriate drug therapy or surgery. Indications for VLCDs are shown in Table 6.2.

Benefits of a VLCD are shown in Table 6.3. Use of an appropriately formulated VLCD in conjunction with an exercise program does not result in an excessive loss of lean body mass. Where VLCDs are combined with an intensive education and support program approximately half of the weight loss remains at 2 years. Even better results can be achieved for the maintenance of weight loss by the addition of medications such as sibutramine or orlistat or with bariatric surgery.

TABLE 6.2
Indications for very-low-calorie diets

When weight reduction is required urgently
- Life-threatening complications
  - respiratory and/or cardiac failure
  - refractory type 2 diabetes
  - severe gastroesophageal reflux disease
- Before elective surgery
  - joint replacement
  - abdominal hernia repair
  - cholecystectomy
  - cardiac surgery
  - before bariatric surgery

When nutritionally complete but low-energy feeding is required for obese patients
- after bariatric surgery
- elderly patients
- ill patients

Where weight reduction will benefit obese subjects who are unable to increase their physical activities because of:
- immobility due to arthritis or neurological disease
- chronic cardiorespiratory disease

Where conventional approaches have failed

Where motivation and/or early demonstrable weight loss is required

VLCDs also reduce comorbidities associated with obesity.
- Reductions in total and LDL cholesterol and triglycerides of approximately 15% may occur; HDL cholesterol decreases in women but increases by about 5% in men.
- Systolic and diastolic blood pressure can be decreased by 8% and 10%, respectively.
- Reversal of the biochemical markers of fatty liver disease result in

77

TABLE 6.3

Advantages of a very-low-calorie diet

- Weight loss of up to 12–20 kg (sometimes more depending on starting weight and adherence) in 8–12 weeks
- Suppression of hunger (related to ketone production)
- Increased sense of well-being (occasionally euphoria)
- Reduced blood pressure
- Improved liver function
- Improved glycemic control
- Improved lung function
- Decrease in gastroesophageal reflux

substantial reductions in liver fat, and non-alcoholic steatohepatitis (NASH) can be reversed.
- In obese patients with type 2 diabetes, blood glucose can often be normalized. In addition, insulin can often be discontinued or the dosage reduced substantially. Dosages of oral hypoglycemics can be reduced by 50–100%.
- Respiratory function (forced expiratory volume in 1 second and forced vital capacity) improves in patients with asthma, accompanied by a reduction in the number of exacerbations and a decrease in the use of oral glucocorticoids.
- Substantial improvements in obstructive sleep apnea occur, with a decrease in the number of desaturation episodes, apneas, hypopneas and arousals.
- The use of VLCDs in patients with Pickwickian syndrome (respiratory and cardiac failure as a result of morbid obesity) achieves rapid and massive weight loss that may prove life-saving.
- This type of diet may also decrease gastroesophageal reflux.
Contraindications for a VLCD are shown in Table 6.4.
Adverse effects. Satisfactorily formulated VLCDs carry negligible short-term risks. Caution should be exercised in patients taking concomitant medication. Doses of hypoglycemics should usually be halved in the first 24 hours of VLCD use in order to avoid

TABLE 6.4

Contraindications for a very-low-calorie diet

- Children and adolescents (< 18 years of age)
- Pregnancy and breastfeeding
- Age > 60–65 years old*
- Eating disorders
- Major depression, bipolar disorder, schizophrenia or substance misuse
- Diabetes mellitus (when oral hypoglycemics or insulin are being used)[†]
- Porphyria

*Unless the clinical indication is compelling, such as severe immobility or cardiorespiratory compromise directly attributable to obesity.
[†]Unless managed by those skilled in the management of obesity, diabetes and with experience in the use of very-low-calorie diets.

hypoglycemia. Because of the large initial diuresis that occurs, caution is required in patients with compromised renal function and in those taking diuretics or digoxin. Clotting function should be closely monitored in patients taking warfarin.

Constipation is common but can be minimized by a high fluid intake and the addition of fiber as described above. Patients with pre-existing hyperuricemia have an increased risk of gout. Gallstones may occur, or may become symptomatic, depending on the rapidity of weight loss. Minor side effects include fatigue, nausea, dizziness, headache, irritability, cold intolerance and bad breath.

Supplemental low-calorie diet or 'modified' VLCD. This approach permits one small meal each day. Commercially available VLCD preparations can be combined with selected foods to provide about 800 kcal per day. For example, 450 kcal/day can be derived from a VLCD and 350 calories from one small meal. This approach promotes adherence by minimizing the disruption of lifestyle activities and facilitating 'social eating'. It is important that added foods are very low in carbohydrate, as consumption of carbohydrate will produce severe

79

hunger and control will almost certainly be lost. An optimal meal might be a small serving (size of the palm of the hand) of meat, fish or chicken with salad or mixed vegetables.

Intermittent use of VLCD. After an initial acute treatment phase of 8–12 weeks, VLCDs can be used on an intermittent basis to maintain the desired weight. Approaches include:

- use of the VLCD for 1–2 weeks every third month
- reintroduction of the VLCD when bodyweight increases to a predetermined level.

Both the 'intermittent' and 'on-demand' approaches result in similar weight loss at 2 years, with concomitant improvement in obesity-related comorbidities. The intermittent use of a VLCD, for example 1 day a week, has been shown to be a useful approach in obese patients with type 2 diabetes, although this remains a controversial area and clearly there are opportunities for further study.

Meal replacements. Another approach is to substitute one or more meals with a sachet of a commercially available VLCD or other nutritionally complete meal replacement. This is often a useful

TABLE 6.5

Key strategies for maintenance of weight loss

People who successfully maintain weight loss for long periods of time without the use of medicines or bariatric surgery:

- consume a moderate-to-low-fat diet (< 30% of total daily caloric intake)
- monitor caloric intake and weight frequently (weekly)
- eat breakfast
- have high levels of physical activity (> 150 minutes' walking or equivalent intentional physical activity per week and at least some resistance exercise every 72 hours; at least some of the time the intensity of the exercise causes shortness of breath)*

*Previously sedentary individuals require expert supervision to attempt this level of intensity.

approach for people who avoid breakfast (which leads to overconsumption later in the day). Use of meal replacements provides structure with portion control and convenience – which are important factors for the maintenance of weight loss (Table 6.5) – and allows prudent additional meals and snacks. In obese subjects, diets with meal replacements have proven more effective than conventional diets. Meal replacements offer a promising strategy for treating obese patients with type 2 diabetes.

Key points – management: diet

- Weight loss requires a negative energy balance, which for most people is achieved more readily by caloric restriction than by increased physical activity.
- Dietary adherence is more important than the specific dietary pattern; choice of diet should therefore consider the particular patient's characteristics in terms of culture, lifestyle, understanding, sex, age etc.
- Important factors in promoting dietary adherence include convenience, choice and an ongoing behavioral support program.
- Healthy diets focus on fruit and vegetables, whole grains and lean unprocessed meat, chicken and seafood. Up to 30% of energy may come from fat but intake of saturated (animal) fat should be very limited. The predominant fats consumed should be of plant origin such as monounsaturated fatty acids (e.g. from olive oil) and long-chain polyunsaturated fatty acids, and omega-3 fatty acids from seafood.
- Sugared beverages should be avoided; water is the ideal drink for hydration.
- Changing to a healthy diet has benefits for cardiometabolic health irrespective of weight loss.

Key references

Bleich SN, Wang YC, Wang Y, Gortmaker SL. Increasing consumption of sugar-sweetened beverages among US adults: 1988–1994 to 1999–2004. *Am J Clin Nutr* 2009;89:372–81.

Ello-Martin JA, Roe LS, Ledikwe JH et al. Dietary energy density in the treatment of obesity: a year-long trial comparing 2 weight-loss diets. *Am J Clin Nutr* 2007;85:1465–77.

Howarth NC, Huang TT, Roberts SB et al. Eating patterns and dietary composition in relation to BMI in younger and older adults. *Int J Obes (Lond)* 2007;31:675–84.

Keogh JB, Clifton PM. The role of meal replacements in obesity treatment. *Obes Rev* 2005;6:229–34.

Livesey G, Taylor R, Hulshof T, Howlett J. Glycemic response and health – a systematic review and meta-analysis: relations between dietary glycemic properties and health outcomes. *Am J Clin Nutr* 2008;87:258–268S.

Raynor HA, Jeffery RW, Ruggiero AM et al. Weight loss strategies associated with BMI in overweight adults with type 2 diabetes at entry into the Look AHEAD (Action for Health in Diabetes) trial. *Diabetes Care* 2008;31:1299–304.

Seagle HM, Strain GW, Makris A et al. Position of the American Dietetic Association: weight management. *J Am Diet Assoc* 2009;109:330–46.

Truby H, Baic S, deLooy A et al. Randomised controlled trial of four commercial weight loss programmes in the UK: initial findings from the BBC "diet trials". *BMJ* 2006;332:1309–14.

Wadden TA, Butryn ML, Wilson C. Lifestyle modification for the management of obesity. *Gastroenterology* 2007;132:2226–38.

For our ancestors, physical activity was a vital element of life, for hunting and to avoid being hunted. Nowadays, however, it has become an annoying intrusion into our comfortable sedentary lives. The modern workforce is much more sedentary, as manual jobs have been mechanized and transport systems and information technology have flourished. Leisure time is also increasingly high-tech and sedentary.

Risks of inactivity

Sedentary behavior and obesity are closely linked but are not necessarily concurrent in the same individual and should be considered as independent risk factors for disease. Inactivity carries a risk even in the lean: lack of physical activity is a risk factor for stroke and coronary artery disease and causes a twofold increase in risk for all-cause mortality, hard on the heels of smoking and hypertension in terms of damage done (Figure 7.1).

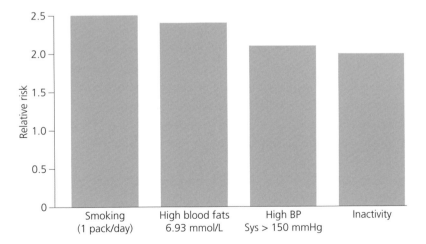

Figure 7.1 Physical inactivity is the fourth primary risk factor for all-cause mortality. Reproduced from Powell et al. 1987 with permission from Annual Reviews.

Benefits of physical activity

Physical activity is an integral and essential part of any long-term weight management program. It:

- improves fitness
- decreases cardiometabolic risk
- helps sustain weight loss
- maintains a lower weight once the initial 5–10% loss has occurred.

A study carried out among Boston policemen showed minimal difference in weight loss with diet alone compared with diet plus exercise whereas the exercise group sustained weight loss in the long term. Other studies have confirmed these findings.

Assessing the clinical benefits of physical activity by weight loss alone is misleading, however. Many studies have shown that the additional weight loss associated with physical exercise is relatively minor compared with diet alone; however, the medical benefits are massive. Regular exercise increases muscle bulk at the expense of fat, thereby increasing the body's fat-free mass. Muscle weighs 1.5 times more than fat, so bodyweight may be maintained or may even increase when patients start performing unaccustomed exercise. The transformation of body morphology is crucial to health: muscle is a much healthier substance than dangerous metabolically active adipose tissue, and also has the advantage of increasing the basal metabolic rate – in contrast to the decrease that usually occurs in patients losing weight – thus aiding concurrent dietary efforts. The waist circumference of someone who becomes fitter by increasing levels of activity will decrease, although their weight may change little. Physical activity also has significant health benefits regardless of whether or not weight loss occurs:

- improved insulin sensitivity, therefore improved control of type 2 diabetes
- improved lipid profile, particularly increased HDL cholesterol
- reduced blood pressure
- improved self-esteem, and reductions in symptoms of depression and anxiety
- improved daily functional capacity
- reduced risk of colorectal cancer because of improved metabolism of environmental carcinogens.

Increasing physical activity is as beneficial to general health as giving up smoking. Individuals who attempt weight loss by physical activity alone should be congratulated on increased fitness, and should be encouraged to monitor their waist circumference, otherwise they may become frustrated and demoralized by lack of change in weight or BMI. Use of bioimpedance analysis to illustrate the changes in body composition may also provide encouragement.

Recommended levels

Current guidelines suggest that to maintain health, an adult should perform a minimum of 30 minutes' moderate physical activity per day in addition to the normal daily routine. This is equivalent to a brisk walk. The 30 minutes can be carried out in one go, or be cumulative over several sessions. Combinations of moderate- and vigorous-intensity activity can be performed to meet this recommendation; for example, the recommendation can be met by walking briskly for 30 minutes twice during the week and jogging for 20 minutes on two other days.

The World Health Organization recommends that 45–60 minutes' of moderate-intensity exercise on most days is necessary to prevent unhealthy weight gain, and 60–90 minutes per day is required to lose weight or prevent weight regain after substantial loss. At least 10 000 steps per day (as monitored on a pedometer) are recommended for health; 15 000 are required to lose weight or maintain weight loss. Extra activity may occur at home, in the gym, park, sports field or shopping center, as long as it is *additional* activity, preferably enjoyable, and likely to be maintained in the long term to avoid rebound weight gain. Every adult should perform activities that maintain or increase muscular strength and endurance a minimum of 2 days each week. Because of the dose–response relation between physical activity and health, people who wish to improve their personal fitness further, reduce their risk for chronic diseases and disabilities or prevent unhealthy weight gain may benefit by doing more than the minimum recommended amounts of physical activity.

Physical activity must be reintroduced to our lives – by scheduled exercise for those who enjoy and can maintain it, or by increasing the amount and quality of activity during the daily routine. Optimally, increases in both types of activity will occur. Figure 7.2 shows that energy expenditure is greatest when physical activity is part of the daily routine, rather than a daily visit to the gym. Individuals with sedentary occupations should ensure that periods of sitting are broken at least every 30 minutes by some form of activity. Strategies to increase incidental activity are shown in Table 7.1.

For the purpose of weight-loss programs, the most effective exercise is aerobic rather than vigorous or explosive exercise. This is partly because of the added cardiovascular risk of unaccustomed severe or strenuous exercise, and partly because aerobic exercise burns off fat stores whereas vigorous anaerobic exercise uses glycogen stores from the liver in preference to fat, which is rapidly replaced by eating carbohydrate after exercise. The optimum degree of 'brisk' exertion

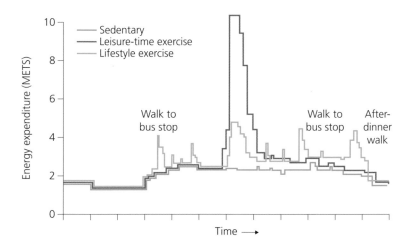

Figure 7.2 Contrasting patterns of energy expenditure over 1 day for a sedentary person (blue line), a person who engages in planned vigorous exercise during leisure time but is otherwise sedentary (red line), and a person with a sedentary job with short bouts of physical activity throughout the day (green line). METS, metabolic equivalent measurement of energy used per kg bodyweight per minute; 1 MET is the energy expenditure at rest, equivalent to 3.3 kcal/kg/hour. Reproduced with permission from Blair SN et al. 1992. © Blackwell Science.

TABLE 7.1

World Health Organization (WHO) recommendations for increasing physical activity

The WHO recommends that energy expenditure is increased by 834 kJ (200 kcal) per day. For the average obese subject, this is equivalent to fidgeting-like activity of 2.5 hours per day or strolling-equivalent activity (1.6–3.2 km/h) of 1 hour per day.

- Identify and help the individual select activities that they will enjoy and that fit into their daily lives.
- Point out that adequate activity is as important and as routine as tooth brushing.
- Broaden the patient's concept of physical activity.
- Identify strategies to incorporate physical activity into everyday life.
- Explore opportunities to be active every day in as many ways as possible.
- Discuss how to be active at home.
- Encourage those patients who are able to undertake some regular vigorous physical activity.
- Focus on sustainable long-term strategies.
- Explore the extent of family support, and identify activities that can be a fun family activity done every day.

quickens the pulse, induces perspiring and quickens the breathing rate but allows a person to talk.

It has been estimated that 75% of adults get less physical activity than they should. One study showed that 56% of men and 52% of women believed they were sufficiently active to benefit health, whereas in fact only 36% and 24%, respectively, achieved even moderate activity. Patients often mistakenly believe they are fit because they manage routine chores without undue tiredness or breathlessness; however, it may be that their daily tasks are too physically mundane to expose their lack of fitness.

Different ethnic groups follow physical activity recommendations to different extents: only 37% of black Caribbean men, 30% of Indian

87

men and 26% of Bangladeshi men were 'sufficiently' active, compared with 37% of the general male population. In women, 11% of Bangladeshi women, 23% of Indian women and 31% of black Caribbean women met the recommendations, compared with 25% of women in the general population.

Individual tailoring. It is important to tailor physical activity recommendations to each individual, setting realistic goals. Any increase in activity levels is important, however little the degree, and induces an almost immediate improvement in insulin sensitivity.

Long-term medical conditions impact on a person's ability to achieve meaningful levels of activity, and appropriate advice must take this into account. For an obese person with chronic bronchitis, a few steps in the garden every hour may represent a significant increase in activity; a patient with asthma may need to be advised to use their salbutamol inhaler before exercising; a slow stroll on even ground may be appropriate for someone with severe vascular disease; advice to stand up while talking on the phone may be helpful for someone with severe physical limitations. The US Surgeon General's report recommends wheeling oneself in a wheelchair for 40 minutes as being a reasonable level of activity for health benefits, whereas a patient with lower-limb orthopedic problems may be advised to perform low-impact activities, or even arm exercises alone. Elderly patients often suffer from sarcopenia, so increased physical activity of any degree should be vigorously promoted for anyone with severe physical limitations.

Children. Armstrong and colleagues demonstrated that almost 50% of girls and 38% of boys did not achieve one 10-minute period of exercise equivalent to brisk walking in 3 school days. The home is safer and more comfortable than ever; children watch an average of almost 3 hours of television per day, often whilst snacking on high-calorie foods, and play computer games with ever increasing complexity, requiring more and more practice to reach the final goal. Gortmaker calculated that the risk of overweight is increased 4.6 times in children who watch more than 5 hours of television per day.

The UK National Audit Office has produced some recommendations to prevent childhood obesity:

- at least 2 hours' physical activity a week for all pupils
- a safer and more integrated network of appropriate routes, footpaths and cycle lanes
- adoption of cycling and walking in preference to traveling by car
- broadening the range of activities schools offer to encourage young people to participate in different forms of physical recreation.

Key points – management: physical activity

- Physical activity is a key component of weight management and is important for maintaining weight lost by any method of treatment.
- Physical activity is beneficial even if weight is lost, as it reduces cardiometabolic risk, insulin resistance and cancer risk.
- Although the amount of weight loss induced by exercise alone may be disappointing, there are beneficial changes in fat distribution and body composition which can be observed by bioimpedance analysis and even waist circumference.
- An increase in physical activity can be achieved by modifications to the daily routine; multiple short bouts are just as beneficial as the equivalent amount of activity performed in one session.
- Some aerobic activity that leads to shortness of breath each day provides additional benefit, and some resistance exercise should also be included.

Key references

American College of Sports Medicine, Chodzko-Zajko WJ, Proctor DN, Fiatarone Singh MA et al. American College of Sports Medicine position stand. Exercise and physical activity for older adults. *Med Sci Sports Exerc* 2009;41:1510–30.

Armstrong N, Balding J, Gentle P, Kirby B. Patterns of physical activity among 11 to 16 year old British children. *BMJ* 1990;301:203–5.

Blair SN, Kohl HW, Gordon NF. Physical activity and health: a lifestyle approach. *Med Exerc Nutr Health* 1992;1;54–7.

Davis JN, Hodges VA, Gillham MB. Physical activity compliance: differences between overweight/obese and normal-weight adults. *Obesity (Silver Spring)* 2006;14:2259–65.

Ehrsam R, Stoffel S, Koerner U et al. Exercise prescription for the overweight and the obese: how to quantify and yet keep it simple. *Br J Sports Med* 2009 Mar 16 (Epub ahead of print).

Gortmaker SL, Must A, Sobol AM et al. Television viewing as a cause of increasing obesity among children in the United States, 1986–1990. *Arch Pediatr Adolesc Med* 1996;150: 356–62.

Haskell WL, Lee IM, Pate RR et al. Physical activity and public health: updated recommendation for adults from the American College of Sports Medicine and the American Heart Association. *Med Sci Sports Exerc* 2007;39:1423–34.

Pavlou KN, Krey S, Steffee WP. Exercise as an adjunct to weight loss and maintenance in moderately obese subjects *Am J Clin Nutr* 1989;49 (5 Suppl):1115–23.

Powell KE, Thompson PD, Caspersen CJ, Kendrick JS. Physical activity and the incidence of coronary heart disease. *Annu Rev Public Health* 1987;8:253–87.

Saris WH, Blair SN, van Baak MA et al. How much physical activity is enough to prevent unhealthy weight gain? Outcome of the IASO 1st Stock Conference and consensus statement. *Obes Rev* 2003;4:101–14.

US Public Health Service. The Surgeon General's call to action to prevent and decrease overweight and obesity 2001. Rockville, MD: US Department of Health and Human Services, 2001. www.surgeongeneral.gov/topics/ obesity/calltoaction/CalltoAction.pdf

8   Management: behavioral therapy

Bringing about a change in behavior is an important part of clinical care; the ability to foster such change in patients is fundamental to the skill base of any healthcare professional. Behavioral therapy – the collective name for the various methods and strategies used to bring about changes in lifestyle – is universally credited as being one of the three main pillars of weight management, alongside dietary modification and increased physical activity, covered in Chapters 6 and 7. Despite its importance, however, behavioral therapy remains something of a mystery to clinicians.

Behavioral therapy for obesity originated in the 1950s and 1960s. The major theory promoted at the time was that obesity was caused by an 'obese eating style' and that therapy would guarantee a return to normal bodyweight by eliminating abnormal eating behavior, and normal weight would therefore be sustained permanently. Although this has clearly not occurred, behavioral techniques have improved. Cognitive behavior therapy (CBT) in particular has an important role in the long-term management of obesity, being key to changing patients' habits and attitudes.

Classic behavioral interventions for managing obese patients may last months or years. However, clinicians can introduce complex behavioral therapy concepts during the course of a normal consultation. In fact, many clinicians do so without realizing, masquerading simply as good advice presented in a logical, ordered fashion. For example, if the first thing an individual does when arriving home from a stressful day is to eat two biscuits, basic dietary and nutritional advice is simple: stop eating biscuits. Behavioral therapy, on the other hand, suggests *how* to avoid eating biscuits: the answer could be simple – don't buy any biscuits – or more complex – avoid the stressful situation that triggered the desire to eat biscuits, which may mean changing jobs, or walking home instead of taking a crowded bus. Other suggestions might include putting the biscuits where they are difficult to reach, and to have healthy snacks such as fruit readily accessible. Alternatively, there may be other ways to unwind: such as having a bath or going for a run.

Behavioral therapy produces disappointing results when used alone, but has much more profound effects when used in combination with other modalities. In short-term studies, it has been shown to induce weight loss of 10% or more but this was not sustained in the long term. However, a long-term support program that combines behavioral therapy with regular physical activity and dietary advice can be highly successful in improving compliance with lifestyle changes and sustaining weight loss.

Stages of change theory

An individual's likelihood of accepting any lifestyle advice depends on their 'stage of change', which refers to the state of mind of an individual and is a reflection of how motivated they are to undergo management for their condition. Before starting treatment it is important to determine which stage the individual is at and to act accordingly; success is unlikely if the wrong approach is made at the wrong time. The six stages are shown in Figure 8.1.

Elements of behavioral therapy

- **Goal setting**: the agreement of realistic weight-loss targets, at a realistic rate of improvement
- **Self-monitoring**: increasing self-awareness of eating patterns and physical activity behavior, which is an essential precursor for change
- **Stimulus control**: avoiding situations that lead to harmful behavior, and promoting situations that influence healthy activity
- **Problem solving**: how to avoid social and societal pressures that might result in straying from agreed goals and targets
- **Cognitive restructuring**: identifying and modifying self-defeating thoughts and ideas.

Many of these techniques are summarized in Table 8.1.

Self-monitoring is a fundamental pillar of CBT; in its most basic form it constitutes a food and activity diary of what is eaten, where and in what circumstances, along with the emotional feelings or triggers involved, and the levels of activity carried out. A food diary should clarify eating patterns and behaviors, particularly events that trigger eating, with a view to changing those patterns once they have been

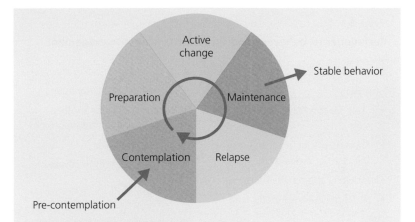

1 **Pre-contemplation:** absolutely no chance of behavioral change in the foreseeable future (i.e. next 6 months)

2 **Contemplation:** awareness that there is a health problem and that something really should be done about it one day (in the next 6 months or so)

3 **Preparation:** awareness is acute and something is going to be done in the next month or so

4 **Active change:** behavior is actively being modified to overcome the problem

5 **Maintenance:** active change has been successful, and consolidation and maintenance are taking place; this phase may last up to 5 years

6 **Stable behavior:** a state of zero temptation – no possibility of returning to old habit.

Note that relapse to an earlier stage can occur at any stage until stage 6 is reached.

Figure 8.1 States of change model. Adapted from Prochaska and DiClemente 1986.

identified, for instance by planning ahead. Once the pattern of eating has been established by recording it in the food diary, the diary can be used as part of the treatment plan, by recording progress towards dietary goals. Long-term weight management has been shown to improve when food records are used.

TABLE 8.1

Techniques of behavior modification for weight management

Stimulus control

Shopping

- Shop for food only on a full stomach
- Shop from a list, and carry only the cash for foods on the list
- Only buy appropriate foods
- Avoid ready-to-eat foods

Plans

- Plan to limit food intake
- Pre-plan meals and snacks
- Substitute exercise for snacking
- Eat meals and snacks at scheduled times
- Don't accept food offered by others

Activities

- Use visual aids to remind yourself to eat properly (pictures, cartoons etc.)
- Make nutritionally acceptable foods attractive to eat
- Remove inappropriate foods from the house or store problem foods out of sight
- Keep healthier foods visible
- Eat all food in the same place
- Remove food from inappropriate storage areas

Serving food

- Keep serving dishes off table
- Use small dishes/utensils
- Avoid being the food server

- Serve/ eat one portion at a time
- Leave the table after eating
- Save leftovers for another meal instead of finishing them

Holidays and parties

- Prepare activities in advance
- Drink less alcohol
- Make eating plan before party
- Eat a low-calorie snack before parties
- Practise polite ways of declining food
- Don't be discouraged by the occasional setback

Self-monitoring

Keep a food diary that includes:

- Time and place of eating
- Type and amount of food
- Who else is present
- How you felt before eating
- Activities that you are doing at the same time
- Calories and/or fat content of foods
- Patterns in your eating

Eating behavior

Slow rate of eating

- Take one small bite at a time; chew well before swallowing
- Put fork down between mouthfuls
- Pause in the middle of the meal and assess hunger

Do nothing else while eating
- Concentrate only on eating
- Focus on enjoying food
- Eat all food in one place
- Follow eating plan

Rewards
- Solicit help from family and friends; ask them to provide praise and material rewards
- Clearly define behaviors to be rewarded
- Utilize self-monitoring records as basis for rewards
- Plan specific rewards for specific behaviors
- Gradually make rewards more difficult to achieve

Nutrition education
- Use food diary to identify problem areas
- Make small changes that can be continued
- Eat a well-balanced diet
- Learn nutritional values
- Decrease fat intake, increase complex carbohydrate intake

Physical activity

Lifestyle activity
- Increase lifestyle activity, including increased use of stairs
- Walk where you would normally use a bus/car
- Record time/frequency/intensity of walking each day

Exercise
- Start a mild exercise program
- Keep a record of daily exercise
- Increase the amount of exercise very gradually

Cognitive restructuring
- Develop realistic expectations of weight loss; set reasonable and realistic weight-loss and behavior-change goals
- Focus on progress, not shortcomings
- Avoid imperatives such as 'always' or 'never'
- Keep a record of thoughts about self and weight; challenge and counter self-defeating thoughts with positive thoughts

Relapse management
- View lapses as opportunities to learn more about behavior change
- Identify triggers for lapsing
- Plan how to prevent lapses
- Generate a list of coping strategies in high-risk situations
- Distinguish hunger from cravings
- Make a list of activities that make it impossible to give in to cravings
- Confront or ignore cravings
- Outlast urges to eat

Adapted from Brownell KD. *The LEARN Program for Weight Management.* American Health Publishing, 2000.

Stimulus control refers to the different stimuli for eating, only one of which is feeling physically hungry. Eating chocolate biscuits on arriving home from work is more likely to be because of stress than hunger; the stimulus control is therefore to remove the biscuit or the stress. Other stimuli for eating are described as 'external cues'; they include:

- time (e.g. eating because its lunchtime)
- presence of food (e.g. eating it because food is available, or finishing a plateful because it is rude or wasteful not to [this can be a habit deeply ingrained from childhood])
- social cues (e.g. eating cheese and biscuits with a glass of port because everyone else is).

Stimulus control might involve avoiding external cues, for instance taking a route home that avoids passing a fast-food outlet. Controlling eating at the last stage of the chain (i.e. when one is already looking at the menu in the window) is incredibly difficult, whereas taking action earlier in the chain, when the meal is less tangible, is easier – take a different route home. Avoiding shopping whilst hungry is another example of stimulus control. Other stimuli such as stress or emotional eating (discussed below) are described as 'internal cues'.

'Learned self-control' becomes important when the only route home passes the fast-food outlet, making external temptation unavoidable. Learned self-control occurs with prolonged repetition of the external stimulus, without giving in and eating. After enough journeys home without buying food, the conditioned response will be reduced.

Problem solving. There is a relationship between high levels of self-efficacy and successful outcomes in obesity management programs. Techniques can be used during a consultation to implement strategies for the management of obesity by using a Problem Solving Therapy (PST) approach. PST facilitates the development of a set of skills that enhance a patient's self-efficacy. Patients are supported to develop the ability to recognize potential solutions to their problems rather than solutions being suggested by the patient's healthcare practitioner. The process is outlined in Table 8.2; the skills developed are transferable to solving a range of problems.

TABLE 8.2

Using problem-solving therapy for the behavioral management of obesity

PST stage	Clinician action
Introduction	• Explain aims and stages • Applicability to many of life's problems • Benefits to be gained in the context of how the patient's life, lifestyle and health is affected
Problem	• Ask the patient to identify the major issues/list current problems • Have them identify which of these they wish to start with today • Discuss the problem with them – let them work through and clarify the various issues surrounding the problem including barriers and facilitators
Goal	• Ask the patient to indicate what they wish to achieve. In formulating the goals with the patient, make sure that they are SMART (specific, measurable, achievable, relevant and timely)
Explore and choose solutions	• Encourage the patient to brainstorm as many solutions as possible and then to consider the pros of cons of each solution and in particular to consider whether a solution will achieve their goal
Implement the solution	• Get the patient to describe their plan to implement the solution. Be sure to include how they will self-monitor, get support from others, and deal with any issues that might derail the plan. Agree on the details of the process and desired outcome
Review (~2 weeks)	• Ask how they got on. If the goal was achieved, encourage and agree on the next target and/or define a new goal and explore solutions. If the goal was not achieved, ask the patient to consider why not, and what changes to the solution might be needed, or whether it might be more appropriate to address other issues

Adapted from Mynors-Wallis L. The seven stages of problem solving treatment. In: *Problem Solving Treatment for Anxiety and Depression*. Oxford: Oxford University Press, 2005. Pierce D, Gunn J. Using problem solving therapy in general practice. *Aust Fam Physician* 2007;36:230–3.

'**Stress management**' is self-explanatory; comfort eating is widely recognized as a reason for overeating. However, evidence for hyperphagia in a stressful environment is conflicting, as for some individuals stress causes loss of appetite. Many people indulge in 'emotional eating': eating at times of stress, pressure or negative emotional state to provide comfort. This amounts to eating without relying on the usual stimulus of hunger to govern when food is required. Such behavior may reflect childhood patterns, even breastfeeding, when eating and comfort were closely associated. Others admit to 'bingeing' on energy-dense foods when commonsense tells them to stop but they feel powerless to resist. These phenomena may arise from common pathways in the brain that relate to satiety and mood; the underlying stress or depression must be confronted for weight loss to be successful.

Eating disorders

Binge eating disorder (BED) is specifically recognized in its own right. Patients with BED display the features of bulimia nervosa but without the purging, abnormal exercise regimens or other compensatory behavior to induce weight loss. The condition was largely ignored when it was first recognized in 1959 but has recently gained greater prominence. Its features include:

- recurrent episodes of eating objectively large amounts of food within a discrete period of time
- a subjective sense of lack of control during each eating episode
- binge eating at least 2 days a week on average for 6 months
- no regular use of inappropriate compensatory behaviors – purging, fasting, excessive exercise.

Binge eating episodes are associated with three or more of the following:

- eating much more rapidly than normal
- eating until feeling uncomfortably full
- eating large amounts of food when not feeling physically hungry
- eating alone because of being embarrassed by how much one is eating
- feeling disgusted with oneself, depressed or guilty after overeating
- marked distress about binge-eating behavior.

It is estimated that 2.5% of adult women and 1.1% of men suffer from BED, most, but not all, of whom are obese. The prevalence among patients attending obesity clinics is 20–30%, emphasizing the importance of recognizing the condition without delay.

Treatment involves conventional weight management combined with CBT. Strict dietary regimens are likely to aggravate the condition and should be avoided. Depression and personality disorders have been linked with BED but it is unclear whether the abnormal eating pattern predates the emotional disorder or vice versa.

Night eating syndrome (NES) was recognized as an abnormal eating pattern in the 1950s by Albert Stunkard, as was its association with psychological and emotional factors. Sufferers tend to be moody, tense, anxious, nervous and depressed; NES is thought to be associated with abnormal reactions to stress and changes in the circadian rhythm, with a disruption of the hypothalamo–pituitary axis. Symptoms and criteria are:

- morning anorexia (i.e. no appetite for breakfast; the first food of the day is delayed by several hours)
- evening hyperphagia (i.e. excess food in the evening – 50% of the day's intake is eaten after the end of the evening meal and after 7 o'clock)
- a pattern of behavior that has persisted for at least 2 months
- guilt feelings whilst eating
- feelings of tension and anxiety but no enjoyment associated with eating
- frequent waking during the night, usually with eating during waking intervals
- consumption of mainly carbohydrates and sugars at inappropriate times
- continuous eating during the evening, unlike BED in which eating is in short episodes.

The prevalence of NES in the general population is 1–2%, rising to 10% of obese patients and as many as a quarter of grossly obese people. It is associated with obstructive sleep apnea and restless legs syndrome, but has no association with nocturnal sleep-related eating disorder, which is more of a sleep disorder than an eating disorder characterized by eating during sleep (rather like sleep walking). Patients with NES lack hunger before their episodes of night eating, display 'automaticity' of the behavior during waking intervals and varying levels of consciousness during eating.

Treatment is predominantly behavioral rather than dietary, initially by persuading patients to have an early substantial breakfast and to regain a normal eating pattern. The circadian rhythm should be reinforced by the appropriate amount of exercise during the day, with normal regular mealtimes and daily routines.

Key points – management: behavioral therapy

- Behavioral therapy, alongside diet and lifestyle advice, is one of the three key components of obesity management.
- A person's degree of motivation and expectations should be assessed.
- Techniques include goal setting, self-monitoring and stimulus control.
- Binge eating disorder and night eating syndrome are specific eating disorders and should be treated accordingly.

Key references

Baker RC, Kirschenbaum DS. Self-monitoring may be necessary for successful weight control. *Behav Ther* 1993;24:377–94.

Ferster CB, Nurnberger JI, Levitt EB. The control of eating. *J Math* 1962;1:87–109.

Kaplan HI, Kaplan HS. The psychosomatic concept of obesity. *J Nerv Ment Dis* 1957;125:181–201.

Mussell MP, Mitchell JE, Weller CL et al. Onset of binge eating, dieting, obesity, and mood disorders among subjects seeking treatment for binge eating disorder. *Int J Eat Disord* 1995;17:395–401.

Prochaska JO, DiClemente CC. Toward a comprehensive model of change. In: Miller WR, Heather N, eds. *Treating Addictive Behaviors: Processes of Change.* New York: Plenum Press, 1986:3–27.

Schenck CH, Mahowald MW. Review of nocturnal sleep-related eating disorders. *Int J Eat Disord* 1994;15:343–56.

Spitzer RL, Yanovski S, Wadden T et al. Binge eating disorder: its further validation in a multisite study. *Int J Eat Disord* 1993;13:137–53.

Wardle J. Treatment of obesity IV: behavioural treatment. In: *Obesity: The Report of the British Nutrition Foundation Task Force.* Blackwell Science, 1999:176–81.

Pharmacological treatments

Pharmacotherapy may be a useful adjunct for the control of bodyweight, inducing a 5–10% greater weight loss than can be achieved with lifestyle measures alone, and is particularly useful for the maintenance of weight loss. Despite considerable effort and investment, however, only two agents have reached, and remain on, the market: orlistat and sibutramine. Rimonabant, a cannabinoid receptor antagonist, was recently withdrawn from the market in Europe following unacceptable problems associated with depression and aggression.

Mechanisms of action. Drugs that are currently available, in development, or have been used to treat obesity can be divided broadly into four main categories (Figure 9.1):
- drugs that work on neurotransmitter systems that modulate food intake or affect energy expenditure or utilization via central and/or peripheral mechanisms; these include:
  - leptin, with its global effects
  - drugs that act at serotonergic and norepinephrinic (noradrenergic) neurons, selectively (fluoxetine and phentermine, respectively), together (sibutramine), or together with dopaminergic-mediated effects (bupropion)
  - endocannabinoid and opioid (naltrexone) system
  - drugs developed primarily as antiepileptic agents that have anorectic effects (zonisamide and topiramate)
- drugs that affect digestion and subsequent absorption of macronutrients (orlistat)
- drugs that affect gastrointestinal neuroendocrine function and gut–brain neural circuitry to alter appetite, satiety and metabolism; some such agents are used in the management of type 2 diabetes and have been shown to produce weight loss (e.g. the amylin receptor agonist pramlintide [licensed in the USA] and glucagon-like peptide [GLP]-1 receptor agonists)

101

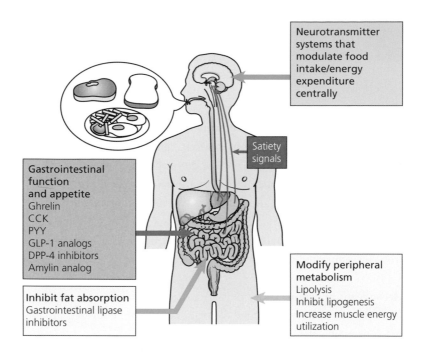

Figure 9.1 Targets for the pharmacological treatment of obesity.
CCK, cholecystokinin; DPP-4, dipeptidyl peptidase 4; GLP-1, glucagon-like
peptide 1; PYY, peptide YY.

- drugs that modify peripheral metabolism by affecting lipolysis,
  lipogenesis or muscle energy utilization.

Currently marketed drugs. Currently only sibutramine and orlistat are
licensed for the long-term management of weight loss. In addition,
phentermine, which has effects on both appetite and energy
expenditure, is available in some countries. Fluoxetine is a selective
serotonin-reuptake inhibitor (SSRI) that may have some benefits in
terms of weight loss in patients with eating disorders.

Sibutramine promotes satiety by inhibiting the reuptake of serotonin
and norepinephrine (noradrenaline), with a secondary effect on energy
metabolism whereby it attenuates some of the decrease in metabolic
rate that follows weight loss. The major side effects are cardiovascular
– hypertension, tachycardia and palpitation – and so regular

monitoring of blood pressure and pulse rate is required. Minor side effects include insomnia, sleep disturbance, nausea, dry mouth and constipation. The usual dose is 10 or 15 mg daily. Sibutramine should not be taken in combination with SSRIs.

Orlistat is a peripherally acting gastric and intestinal lipase inhibitor that reduces fat digestion and absorption. Side effects relate to the gastrointestinal system and include oily spotting, flatus with discharge, fecal urgency, fatty/oily stool, oily evacuation, increased defecation and occasionally fecal incontinence. These effects are proportional to the fat content of the diet and so may encourage patients to reduce the amount of fat they consume. They may also, however, have an adverse effect on compliance, with patients avoiding medication if they are planning to consume a high-fat meal. The usual dose of orlistat is 120 mg three times daily and it must be taken with meals.

Phentermine, which is not available in Europe but is used in the USA and other parts of the world, is a norepinephrine-releasing agent. Phentermine is effective in producing short-term weight loss but there are no data on long-term benefits. Central nervous system, gastrointestinal and genitourinary effects may occur. The most common reported reactions are palpitations, tachycardia and hypertension. Cardiovascular and cerebrovascular events have been described, and potential risks include valvular heart disease and primary pulmonary hypertension. The drug should not be taken in combination with SSRIs.

Fluoxetine is an SSRI that has a mild and poorly sustained impact on weight but is sometimes used in high doses in patients with bulimia or binge eating disorder. Depression is frequent in patients with obesity and requires specific management in order to effectively implement a weight management program. Fluoxetine and other SSRIs are the drugs of choice in this situation because, at worst, they have a neutral effect on weight.

Matching the patient with the drug: appropriate use of pharmacotherapy. There are no clear guidelines for the choice of agent for a particular patient. In general, centrally acting agents produce a more marked benefit than those with a purely peripheral mechanism of action. Orlistat and sibutramine produce clinically meaningful weight loss in significant numbers of patients, beyond that achieved with lifestyle modification alone. However, coadministration has no benefits over either drug alone. The effects on obesity-related comorbidities differ between patient groups, and are difficult to compare directly without matched patient populations. Each drug has a different side-effect profile; the choice of drug should therefore reflect the underlying metabolic and cardiovascular risk profile of the patient and the contraindications to the use of each agent by a given patient. In addition, it is important to consider the individual needs or preferences of the patient. Recent work on the 'psychological profiling' of the drugs suggests that it may be possible to target specific drugs to the patient's personality: patients with personality traits that imply order and conscientiousness may do better with orlistat whereas patients with little control over their eating habits may respond better to the satiety-enhancing properties of sibutramine.

Weight-loss drugs should only be used as part of a comprehensive weight management program, as this is when they are most effective. In one study of a comprehensive behavioral program combined with sibutramine treatment, 52% of patients lost more than 10% of their weight and maintained the loss at 1 year, and 73% lost more than 5% at 1 year. For many patients, the modest weight loss associated with the use of these medications may seem disappointing, leading to frustration and limiting compliance with the overall weight management program. In order to avoid this, it is essential at the outset that clinicians spend time counseling patients and managing their expectations. The aim should be to improve well-being and reduce cardiometabolic risk. It has been shown that modest weight loss induced by orlistat can reduce the incidence of diabetes mellitus over and above that achieved by lifestyle modification alone. It is not known whether weight loss with sibutramine confers any particular benefit. The outcomes in terms of cardiovascular events and a reduction in overall mortality will be known once the outcome of the large multicenter Sibutramine and Cardiovascular Outcomes Trial (SCOUT) is known. Sibutramine and orlistat have been shown to be most effective when used for maintenance of weight loss, rather than induction.

Efficacy of pharmacotherapy for weight loss and maintenance of weight loss. Orlistat induces less weight loss than sibutramine: over a 4-year period, orlistat produced a 3 kg greater weight loss and better maintenance of weight loss than an intensively administered lifestyle program alone. With sibutramine, responders in the Sibutramine Trial of Obesity Reduction and Maintenance (STORM) maintained about 5 kg greater weight loss than achieved with lifestyle alone.

Impact on metabolic and cardiovascular risk factors. Whereas obese patients tend to place most importance on the degree of weight loss that they can, or plan to, achieve, the treating clinician is more concerned with the impact of weight loss on the patient's metabolic and cardiovascular risk profile.

The effects of the different weight-loss agents on these various metabolic factors depend on the individual patient's baseline levels of risk and the magnitude of weight lost, together with any possible drug effects that may be independent of weight loss, all of which make comparisons between studies complex.

Type 2 diabetes. Patients with higher baseline plasma glucose levels have a greater improvement in glycemic control. Both sibutramine and orlistat produce greater reductions in HbA_{1c} than placebo. Pooled data indicate a reduction in HbA_{1c} of approximately 0.5% at 1 year; orlistat has a greater effect than sibutramine.

Lipids. Sibutramine and orlistat have different effects on the fasting lipid profile. Sibutramine reduces triglycerides and raises HDL cholesterol but has no effect on LDL cholesterol. Orlistat provides smaller reductions in triglycerides and significant reductions in LDL cholesterol but with a neutral or small effect on HDL cholesterol. Across the orlistat trials, there appears to be a specific effect on LDL cholesterol beyond that seen with weight loss alone. Changes in HDL cholesterol levels in trials of sibutramine seemed to be more than would be expected from the amount of weight lost.

Blood pressure. Effects on blood pressure are important considerations in relation to pharmacotherapy. The Cochrane meta-analysis showed a mean increase in systolic blood pressure with sibutramine of 1.9 mmHg relative to placebo and in diastolic blood pressure of 1–4 mmHg over 52 weeks, while for orlistat both systolic and diastolic blood pressure decreased over 52 weeks. However, the pattern of effects is different when the data are stratified by weight-loss category rather than considering mean data irrespective of weight change. For example, in a meta-analysis of studies conducted in 4636 patients treated with sibutramine and 2255 placebo recipients, stratifying the change in blood pressure by weight loss indicated a small increase in blood pressure among patients who did not lose weight or who lost less than 5% of their initial bodyweight. However, patients who achieved weight loss of 5% or more showed a decrease in blood pressure that correlated with the decline in weight, although this was slightly attenuated compared with subjects who achieved such a weight loss by diet alone.

Emerging concepts in pharmacotherapy. Although the combination of orlistat and sibutramine is no better than either drug alone, a number of preliminary clinical trials have shown that combining agents with different mechanisms of action allows lower doses of each to be used, with a commensurate reduction in side effects but an additive effect for weight reduction. Moreover, early experience with three-drug combinations produced weight loss of a magnitude approaching that achieved with surgery. Examples of combinations being investigated are topiramate and phentermine; naltrexone and bupropion; bupropion and zonisamide, and pramlintide and leptin.

Bariatric surgery

'Bariatric surgery' refers to surgical procedures that lead directly to weight loss, used in the management of obesity and related comorbidities. The surgical treatment of obesity is a vital (and cost-effective) facet of weight management, and may be the only effective means by which certain individuals can lose significant amounts of weight. Recent technological advances in surgical techniques have led to safer, better and cheaper operations, so although the surgical option is still limited to a relatively small number of extremely obese people, for such patients it can be a vital means of improving health and quality of life.

Historically, two categories of bariatric surgery procedures were performed: restrictive and malabsorptive, which were used either alone or in combination.

Malabsorptive surgery involves reducing the functional length of bowel through which the food passes, so that less of the ingested food is absorbed from the gut. Postoperatively, patients can eat what they please but unabsorbed nutrients pass through the bowel.

Gastric (Roux-en-Y) bypass surgery is a commonly used first-line procedure. A segment of stomach is surgically isolated from the rest and anastomosed to the proximal jejunum, bypassing the majority of the stomach and the entire duodenum (Figure 9.2). This has the advantage of restricting food intake but also induces a degree of malabsorption. This technique induces and maintains long-term weight loss because of its combined approach, but it is a bigger and more

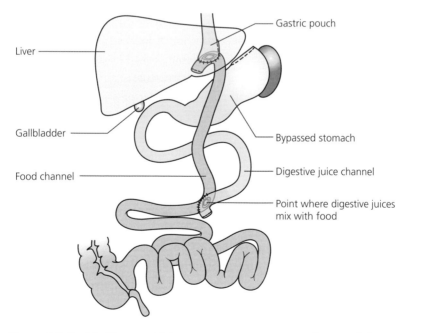

Figure 9.2 Gastric (Roux-en-Y) bypass surgery: a segment of stomach is surgically isolated from the rest and anastomosed to the proximal jejunum, bypassing the majority of the stomach and the entire duodenum.

technically challenging procedure than gastroplasty (see below). Malabsorption, especially of iron, folate and vitamin B_{12} can occur postoperatively, requiring careful monitoring.

Jejuno–ileal bypass has not been performed since about 1980, although individuals who had the operation in the 1970s or earlier may still present. About 90% of the small bowel was bypassed by attaching the top of the jejunum to the end of the ileum, effectively reducing the capacity of the bowel to only about 45 cm, causing rapid transit of food through the bowel and therefore inadequate digestion, malabsorption and steatorrhea. The aim of allowing patients to eat and drink without dietary restrictions but to still lose weight was successful, but the procedure caused an unacceptable incidence of severe, potentially life-threatening complications and side effects such as acute hepatic failure, cirrhosis, oxalate nephropathy, chronic renal failure, immune complex arthritis and malabsorption syndromes.

Restrictive surgery reduces the functional size of the stomach so that smaller quantities of food induce a feeling of fullness. Food eaten in excess of this amount can result in discomfort or bloating and may be regurgitated or vomited. Examples of restrictive surgery include gastric stapling and laparoscopic gastric banding. After passing through the restricted portion of the stomach, food passes through the rest of the bowel, ensuring that nutrients are absorbed normally.

Gastroplasty involves partitioning a 15–40 mL pouch at the top of the stomach (Figure 9.3). This rapidly fills with food and empties slowly through a narrow canal into the body of the stomach, restricting the volume of food eaten. The vertical banded gastroplasty was the forerunner to the laparoscopic gastric band, which involves wrapping an adjustable band around the top of the stomach to reduce functional capacity. The degree of restriction can be manipulated by the surgeon (but not the patient) by increasing or decreasing the pressure through a subcutaneous epigastric or abdominal port. The restrictive procedures have the advantages of lower cost, technical ease, low surgical risk and the absence of any long-term malabsorption. The disadvantages, as demonstrated by the Swedish Obese Subjects (SOS) study described below, is that the degree of sustained weight loss is likely to be less than

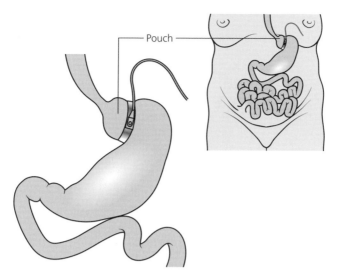

Pouch

Figure 9.3 Laparoscopic gastric banding. The pouch created at the top of the stomach rapidly fills with food and empties slowly through a narrow passage into the larger remainder of the stomach. The band can be tightened or loosened over time to change the size of the passage.

with other procedures. Patients may discover that high-calorie liquids such as milkshakes, melted ice-cream and alcohol pass rapidly through the stoma without causing the sensation of fullness or discomfort, thus minimizing the effects of surgery.

Other surgical procedures

'Superobesity'. More drastic forms of surgery can be used for so-called 'superobese' individuals who have a BMI greater than 50 kg/m², who are 225% overweight or weigh more than 180 kg (400 lb) with life-threatening obesity-related morbidity. Procedures involve resecting the distal 80% of the stomach, with gastro–ileostomy and diversion of biliary and pancreatic secretions to the distal ileum (Figure 9.4). This results in intense weight loss with malabsorption, especially of the fat-soluble vitamins, folate, vitamin B_{12}, iron and calcium, all of which need monitoring and often supplementing.

Artificial bezoar. This is a balloon that is inflated in the stomach, restricting the residual volume of the organ and hence food intake. It is

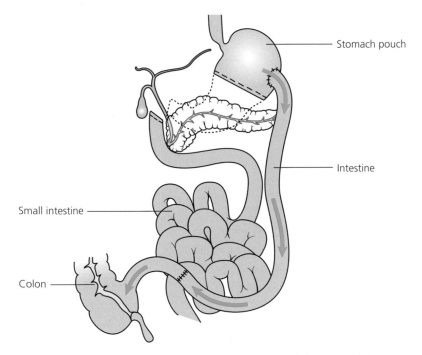

Figure 9.4 Biliopancreatic diversion. The distal 80% of the stomach is resected and the small pouch that remains is connected directly to the final segment of the small intestine, completely bypassing the duodenum and the jejunum.

sometimes used when weight loss is urgent and critical, but has no use in long-term programs.

Gastric pacing devices are being studied for their effects on weight loss; a laparoscopically implanted device is inserted into the stomach wall, stimulation of which induces satiety in a patient.

Skin contouring. Apronectomy is performed after dramatic weight loss to remove overhanging folds of excess skin. Other skin contouring operations include brachioplasty, and the inner and outer aspects of the thighs. Men may undergo correction of pseudogynecomastia.

Liposuction, which involves suction of subcutaneous fat via a trochar, can remove up to 12 liters of fat in extreme cases. This procedure is purely cosmetic and has no impact on the cardiometabolic risk conferred by visceral fat.

Jaw wiring is an obsolete procedure – even if successful, weight lost was rapidly regained on removal of the wires.

Success rates. Bariatric surgery is extremely successful in inducing long-term weight loss because the intervention is almost always permanent, reducing the risk of rebound weight gain. Reductions in excess bodyweight of 50–60% or a decrease in BMI of 10 kg/m² can be expected during the 12–24 months after surgery. Thus, a person weighing 135 kg (300 lb) might realistically expect to lose about 44 kg (100 lb).

The SOS cohort study is the highest profile study of bariatric surgery, and possibly of any branch of the study of obesity. It was started in 1987 and included over 4000 patients, who either underwent substantial weight loss by bariatric surgery or remained weight stable by conventional non-surgical management. Its primary aim was to examine whether total mortality is reduced when obese subjects intentionally lose weight; secondary aims were to study the effects of weight loss on specific mortality and morbidity factors such as cardiovascular disease and diabetes, as well as health-related quality of life and health economics.

Figure 9.5 shows weight loss induced over a 10-year period in a control group who received the conventional treatment and groups who underwent gastric banding, vertical banded gastroplasty (now obsolete) or gastric-bypass procedures. Maximum weight loss in all three surgical groups occurred after 1 year. After 10 years, 4% of control patients had lost more than 20% of their original weight, compared with 74% of the patients in the gastric bypass group. By contrast, weight loss of less than 5% was seen in 73% of controls but 25% of the group that underwent roux-en-Y bypass, the most successful group. The true success of the study, however, is demonstrated by the corresponding cardiometabolic improvements, shown in Figure 9.6.

In other studies, type 2 diabetes has been shown to resolve in 90% of patients, and hypertension in two-thirds, with improvements in HDL cholesterol, total cholesterol and triglycerides. Cardiovascular parameters also improve, including left ventricular wall thickness and left ventricular function. Pulmonary function improves and symptomatic

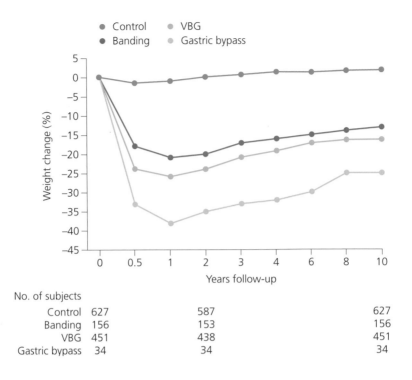

No. of subjects

Control	627	587	627
Banding	156	153	156
VBG	451	438	451
Gastric bypass	34	34	34

Figure 9.5 Weight loss following bariatric surgery among patients who completed 10 years of study in the Swedish Obese Subjects study. Average weight change in the total group of surgically treated patients was almost identical to that in the VBG subgroup. VBG, vertical banded gastroplasty. Reprinted from Rydén A, Torgerson JS. *Surg Obes Relat Dis* 2006;2:549–60 with permission from Elsevier.

obstructive sleep apnea (OSA) can disappear. Table 9.1 shows rates of remission and improvement in another study in which 295 participants underwent laparoscopic adjustable silicone gastric banding. Over a mean period of 44 months' follow-up, patients showed improvement in stress incontinence, OSA, peripheral edema and regulation of menstruation. Greater weight loss was associated with better reduction in arthralgia and dyspnea, and improvements in self-esteem and physical performance.

The chances of developing comorbidities are also reduced by surgery; individuals who have undergone surgery are less likely to develop type 2

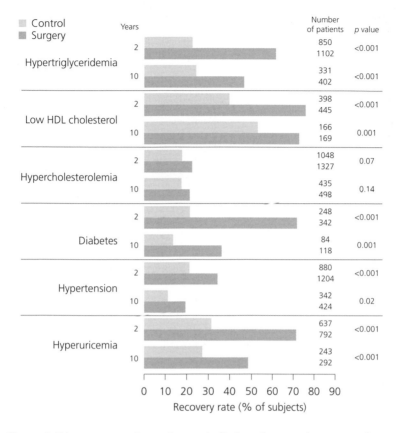

Figure 9.6 Improvement in cardiometabolic function 2 and 10 years after bariatric surgery in the Swedish Obese Subjects study. *p* values were adjusted for sex, age and body mass index at study inclusion. HDL, high-density lipoprotein. Reprinted from Rydén A, Torgerson JS. *Surg Obes Relat Dis* 2006;2:549–60 with permission from Elsevier.

diabetes at both 2 and 8 years or hypertension at 2 years than those who have had non-surgical intervention.

Indications. Unless morbidly obese (see below), a patient is unlikely to be considered for bariatric surgery until they have undergone treatment by diet, lifestyle changes, behavioral therapy and usually drug therapy. The US National Institutes of Health (NIH) criteria for selecting patients for bariatric surgery are given in Table 9.2.

TABLE 9.1

Rate of remissions and improvement in comorbidities following adjustable gastric banding

	Remission (% of patients)	Improvement (% of patients)
Diabetes	75	8
Hypertension	58	42
Dyspnea	85	12
Arthralgia	52	24
Esophageal reflux	79	11
Self-esteem	45	39
General physical functioning	58	33

Data from Frigg et al. 2004.

TABLE 9.2

Criteria established by the US National Institutes of Health for selecting patients for bariatric surgery

- Patient has failed non-surgical attempts to lose weight for at least 5 years; documentation of such attempts should be provided at the time of consultation (if unavailable, a medically supervised weight reduction program may be recommended before bariatric surgery is considered)
- Patient is more than 100 lbs (44 kg) overweight or twice their ideal weight
- Patient fully understands the importance of the proposed surgical procedure, including all known and unknown risks
- Patient is willing to be observed for a prolonged period of time

Patients with morbid obesity (also referred to as 'clinically severe obesity' or 'extreme obesity') are eligible for bariatric surgery using the criteria drawn up by the 1991 NIH Consensus Conference Statement on Gastrointestinal Surgery for Severe Obesity. This constitutes a BMI of at least 40 kg/m^2 or of at least 35 kg/m^2 in the presence of high-risk comorbid conditions. These criteria are widely recognized and accepted. However, recent guidelines developed by the UK National Institute for Health and Clinical Excellence (NICE) state that individuals with a BMI above 50 kg/m² should be offered bariatric surgery as a first-line treatment. For all other patients, weight reduction surgery can only be considered when non-surgical measures have failed.

Other authorities use a broader definition; a strictly weight-based definition is sometimes not appropriate, and a better definition of morbid obesity includes patients who have direct weight-related serious morbidity, such as mechanical arthropathy, hypertension, type 2 diabetes, lipid-related cardiovascular disease and OSA.

Despite the existence of formal guidelines that deem surgery to be an appropriate procedure for patients with morbid obesity, even in the USA, where bariatric surgery is relatively common, only 0.6% of an estimated 11.5 million morbidly obese patients in 2002 underwent bariatric procedures. However, the numbers more than quadrupled between 1998 and 2002 – from 13 386 to 71 733—including a 900% increase in procedures on patients between the ages of 55 and 64 years.

Children and adolescents. Bariatric surgery in childhood and adolescence is controversial, but is now being recommended in extreme cases by authorities such as the National Health and Medical Research Council in Australia. The American Heart Association (AHA) guidelines recommend that bariatric surgery is reserved for full-grown adolescents with the severest obesity-related morbidity:

- BMI above 40 kg/m² and severe associated comorbidities such as OSA, type 2 diabetes or pseudotumor cerebri
- survival treatment when BMI is above 50 kg/m² in the presence of less severe comorbidities such as hypertension and dyslipidemia, particularly if the degree of overweight hinders activities of daily living.

The AHA guidelines underline the critical importance of a comprehensive medical and psychological evaluation, performed by a multidisciplinary team, for selection of appropriate candidates, and the need for sophisticated and often intense postoperative care. The AHA also points out that short-term mortality appears to be low but significant complications can occur. Information on intermediate and long-term outcomes, including malabsorption of critical nutrients, is lacking.

Presurgical assessment. Intensive screening should be carried out before surgery, including evaluation of biochemical and endocrine function. Psychological assessment is particularly important, as bariatric surgery can have huge pyschological effects, but is largely irreversible. This is described in more detail below.

Mental health problems are highly prevalent in grossly obese patients, including eating disorders, depression, low self-esteem and suicidal ideas. It is essential to diagnose and treat such conditions before embarking on surgery, redirecting patients to alternative channels of therapy as needed. Postoperative problems often result from pre-existing depressive disorders not resolving as anticipated; such problems should be addressed beforehand. Conditions such as binge eating disorder and night eating syndrome (see Chapter 8) should be managed before considering surgery. Some psychiatric conditions (see below) are absolute contraindications for bariatric surgery.

The risk:benefit ratio must be considered individually for each patient before surgery, and patients may be deemed unsuitable for surgery depending on their comorbidities and anesthetic risk.

Contraindications. Schizophrenia, personality disorder, uncontrolled depression and other serious mental illnesses are absolute contraindications for surgery.

Women of childbearing age should only undergo surgery after careful consideration, because the increased nutritional needs of pregnancy would be compromised by the reduced capacity for absorption. Women should be strongly urged to use contraception after surgery until their weight has stabilized and their micronutrient status has been checked.

Surgical risk. In major trials a small number of deaths occurred as a result of surgical complications. Perioperative problems include subphrenic abscess (7%), pneumonia (4%), wound infection (4–6%), pulmonary complications (3–6%) and hepatic dysfunction (1.5%). In 2002, in-hospital death rates among patients undergoing weight-loss surgery were 0.32%; the rate was three times higher in men than in women.

Obesity, particularly morbid obesity, is itself a risk factor for surgery, adding significantly to the perioperative complication rate, whatever the procedure. Obese patients are four times more likely to develop perioperative respiratory events, and morbid obesity is linked with adverse respiratory events including pulmonary atelectasis during anesthesia.

Renal clearance of drugs is faster because of increased renal blood flow and glomerular filtration rate; calculating drug dosages in obese patients is complex. Furthermore, drugs such as benzodiazepines and barbiturates are highly lipophilic, which also complicates prescribing. Opioids are avoided if possible, because of unreliable absorption from intramuscular and subcutaneous routes and the risk of respiratory depression.

Peripheral and central access can be hampered by excess fat at cannulation sites, and intubation may be hazardous because of excess cervical fat and palatal and pharyngeal soft tissue.

Postoperatively, the risks of skin infections, pressure sores, aspiration pneumonitis, deep venous thrombosis and sudden death from pulmonary embolism are also raised in obese individuals.

Long-term adverse effects. The most common adverse effects after bariatric surgery are vomiting and feelings of bloating and stomach distension after eating. Malabsorptive procedures can lead to deficiency of iron, vitamin B_{12} and other vitamins, and dumping syndrome (symptoms such as cramps, nausea, diarrhea and dizziness that occur when food or liquid enter the small intestine too quickly) is relatively common.

Psychological implications. Bariatric surgery can have huge psychological implications for the individual.
- The patient will be unable to eat a meal above a certain size, or to eat certain foods without discomfort.
- The patient may have difficulty coming to terms with the loss of the capacity to eat and drink freely, or go out for a meal without risking the unwanted side effects of discomfort and vomiting.
- The patient will experience changes in body image and self-esteem.
- The way the patient is viewed by their spouse, friends, relatives and the public will also change.

Some patients are so desperate to lose weight at any cost that they do not give much thought to 'life after surgery'. Counseling is vital to discuss the patient's expectations and to ensure that they understand the likely reality, and that they have the temperament and psychological stability to deal with the ramifications of surgery.

Whilst undergoing conservative treatment, a patient can choose whether to turn up to their weight management class, whether to walk or drive, whether to give in to desires to eat or whether to take their weight-loss drug. However, by deciding to undergo bariatric surgery, an individual is essentially surrendering control of their weight to another person, and a permanent change takes place. For some patients this handing over of responsibility amounts to an admission of failure, whereas others view it as a great opportunity. Some individuals see it as a chance to deflect the blame onto someone else if they still fail to lose weight.

Both primary and secondary care teams have a responsibility to ensure that a patient considering bariatric surgery is aware of the profound changes that are in store and that they are adequately prepared, and to provide care and support, both physically and psychologically, after surgery.

A growing role for primary care. Many primary care professionals are not well versed in the surgical management of obesity and do not know enough about the procedures available and their sequelae to offer adequate support to patients. The advent of laparoscopic techniques heralds a likely increase in the number of procedures performed, but surgical centers already have severely limited time for perioperative counseling. Primary care practitioners will therefore assume a more significant role in providing preoperative, postoperative, medium- and long-term advice and support. They should convey to a patient the permanent nature of the surgery and realistic expectations: that they will probably lose about 50% of their excess weight but may still consider themselves overweight once their condition stabilizes. They also need to be aware of which patients are suitable for surgery and what the operative criteria are.

Key points – pharmacological and surgical treatments

- Pharmacotherapy should only be used as an adjunct to lifestyle modification.
- Pharmacotherapy is more effective for the maintenance than induction of weight loss but must be used on an ongoing basis for maintenance of effect.
- Pharmacotherapy with orlistat or sibutramine improves the cardiovascular risk factors associated with obesity.
- Orlistat has been shown to be safe and effective, and to prevent the onset of type 2 diabetes mellitus, over a 4-year period.
- Bariatric surgery is among the most clinically effective and cost-effective procedures in medicine.
- The majority of cases of diabetes resolve after surgery.
- Adjustable gastric banding and Roux-en-Y bypass are performed laparoscopically.

Key references

Anon. Randomised trial of jejunoileal bypass versus medical treatment in morbid obesity. The Danish Obesity Project. *Lancet* 1979;2:1255–8.

Chung F, Mezei G, Tong D. Pre-existing medical conditions as predictors of adverse events in day-case surgery. *Br J Anaesth* 1999;83:262–70.

Elfhag K, Rössner S, Barkeling B, Rooth P. Sibutramine treatment in obesity: initial eating behaviour in relation to weight loss results and changes in mood. *Pharmacol Res* 2005;51:159–63.

Encinosa WE, Bernard DM, Steiner CA, Chen CC. Use and costs of bariatric surgery and prescription weight-loss medications. *Health Aff (Millwood)* 2005;24:1039–46.

Frigg A, Peterli R, Peters T et al. Reduction in co-morbidities 4 years after laparoscopic adjustable gastric banding. *Obes Surg* 2004;14:216–23.

NICE. *Obesity: Guidance on the Prevention, Identification, Assessment and Management of Overweight and Obesity in Adults and Children.* CG43. London: National Institute for Health and Clinical Excellence, 2006. www.nice.org.uk/nicemedia/pdf/CG43 NICEGuideline.pdf

Norris SL, Zhang X, Avenell A et al. Pharmacotherapy for weight loss in adults with type 2 diabetes mellitus. *Cochrane Database Syst Rev* 2005;1:CD004096. www.thecochranelibrary.com

Padwal R, Li SK, Lau DC. Long-term pharmacotherapy for obesity and overweight. *Cochrane Database Syst Rev* 2004;3:CD004094. www.thecochranelibrary.com

Torgerson JS, Hauptman J, Boldrin MN, Sjöström L. XENical in the prevention of diabetes in obese subjects (XENDOS) study: a randomized study of orlistat as an adjunct to lifestyle changes for the prevention of type 2 diabetes in obese patients. *Diabetes Care* 2004;27:155–61.

Wadden TA, Berkowitz RI, Womble LG et al. Randomized trial of lifestyle modification and pharmacotherapy for obesity. *N Engl J Med* 2005;353:2111–20.

Children

Prevalence. The prevalence of childhood obesity is increasing throughout the developed world. Figure 10.1 shows the ubiquitous increase in childhood obesity across Europe, and also the alarming dog-leg that represents the recent acceleration in levels in the UK. Rates as high as 55% overweight and obese children in Malta and 36% in Southern Italy have been reported. Figure 10.2 demonstrates the situation in the USA.

The prevalence of obesity among children aged 2–10 years in the UK rose from 10% to 14% between 1995 and 2003 and was most marked among children aged 8–10 years, rising from 11% in 1995 to 17% in 2003. The recent (2008) National Child Measurement Programme found that 22.9% of year 1 primary school children

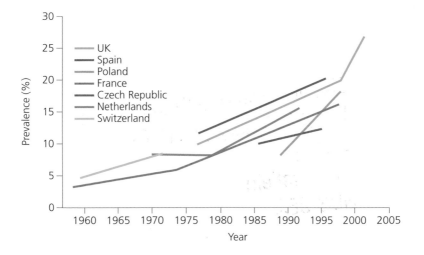

Figure 10.1 The prevalence of overweight/obesity in children and adolescents in Europe is increasing rapidly. More than 80 million European children and adolescents are now overweight or obese. Adapted from *Obesity in Europe: The Case for Action. IOTF/EASO*, 2002, and IOTF data, 2004.

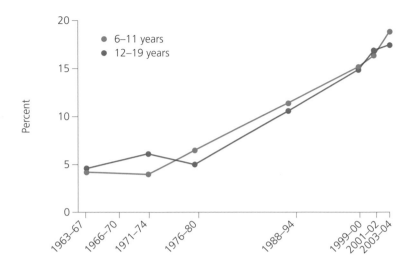

Figure 10.2 Trends in childhood and adolescent overweight in the USA. Overweight is defined as BMI ≥ sex- and weight-specific 95th percentile from the 2000 CDC growth charts. Sources: National Health Examination Surveys II (ages 6–11) and III (ages 12–17), National Health and Nutrition Examination Surveys I–III and 1993–2004.

(aged 5–6 years) were overweight or obese. However, recent data from Western Europe, the UK and Australia suggest that a plateau may have been reached.

Implications of childhood obesity. Three-quarters of obese children go on to become obese adults, carrying their risk factors and comorbidities with them as they grow. The remaining 25% have a 'shadow' cast over their future adult health, because of the metabolic and pathophysiological changes that start early in life. Specialist centers are already reporting comorbidities such as type 2 diabetes – formally known as 'maturity-onset' diabetes – occurring prematurely in children, up to a quarter of whom fulfil the criteria for the metabolic syndrome. Other weight-related illnesses now being seen in childhood include hypertension and dyslipidemia in children as young as 9, and left ventricular hypertrophy. A quarter of children between the ages of 4 and 10 with a BMI greater than the 95th centile have impaired glucose tolerance, 4% have frank type 2 diabetes and 25% have clinical hypertension. Postmortem studies on obese children who died from unrelated causes have revealed atherosclerosis and coronary artery disease. The catastrophic effects of early-onset type 2 diabetes are demonstrated by the Winnipeg Study which identified all the obese adolescents under 17 years of age in the Winnipeg area who had been diagnosed with diabetes by 1986, and followed their progress until 2002. The observation revealed that amongst the 86 children fulfilling the criteria there were:

- two deaths, at ages 25 and 31 years
- one toe amputation at age 26
- three on renal dialysis, at ages 26, 28 and 29 (the 26 year old was also blind)
- 35 live offspring among 56 pregnancies.

Obesity in children also leads to worsening of asthma, obstructive sleep apnea (OSA), slipped epiphyseal plates and Blount's disease of the tibia, and gallstones, as well as profound psychological repercussions and discrimination.

Causes. Childhood obesity is caused by the obesogenic environment described on page 29 – sedentary behavior and unhealthy eating.

A child's natural inclination is to be active, but the modern developed world offers more instantly gratifying sedentary pursuits: computer games that require hours of dedicated practice to 'win'; televisions with a plethora of channels to view, which many children can watch on their own set in their bedroom. More children are being driven to school than ever before, under the pretext of safety and convenience. Children are being conditioned to be inactive from infancy.

Children's eating habits reflect those of adults, compounded by the promotion of unhealthy foods to children.

Parents are notoriously poor at recognizing obesity in their offspring, and it is becoming increasingly difficult as mean childhood BMI increases and there are fewer 'normal' peers for comparison. Without recognition of obesity there is no motivation for change in lifestyle, without which there is no effective answer to childhood obesity.

Assessment should include:

- personal and family history of obesity and related conditions
- physical activity and eating patterns
- psychological factors: bullying, abuse, depression, bereavement, eating disorders
- academic and social progress.

Examination should include height, weight and BMI. BMI is still considered to be the best measure of adiposity in children and adolescents (although this is arguable). Currently available BMI charts show the centiles for boys and girls and the levels of BMI at each age that correspond to the adult categories of overweight and obese.

Urinalysis should be carried out routinely, but other investigations such as blood pressure measurement (with an appropriate-sized cuff) and blood tests only if prompted by abnormal findings in the history or examination.

Specialist referral may be indicated in severe or resistant cases:

- serious morbidity related to obesity (e.g. OSA, orthopedic problems, diabetes mellitus, hypertension)
- height below 9th centile, unexpectedly short for family, or slowed growth velocity
- precocious (before 8 years) or late puberty (no signs at age 13 years in girls, age 15 years in boys)
- significant learning disability
- symptoms/signs of genetic or endocrine abnormalities
- severe and progressive obesity before 2 years of age
- other significant concerns.

Treatment. The burden of treating obesity is borne by the medical profession, and is an onerous one. In treating childhood obesity, just as in adult obesity, it is important to identify individuals who are likely to benefit most from valuable time and resources; success relies on the motivation of the child and family. Successful weight management is usually impossible without a stable and motivated family environment. Ideally, improvements in lifestyle introduced for the benefit of a child will allow the child to act as a catalyst for change within the entire family.

MEND is a community, family-based multidisciplinary program for overweight and obese children aged between 7 and 12 years and their families. It places equal emphasis on (M)ind, (E)xercise, (N)utrition and (D)iet (although the 'D' now stands for 'do it!'), combining all the elements known to be vital in treating and preventing overweight or obesity in children, including family involvement, practical education in nutrition and diet, increasing physical activity and behavioral change. The MEND program is described in more detail on page 137.

Guidelines developed by the UK Royal College of Paediatric and Child Health (RCPCH) and the National Obesity Forum (NOF) recommend a combination of healthy eating, weight management and increased physical activity, as detailed below.

Weight management. It is unusual to advise weight loss in a child, except in extreme cases. The usual weight management goals are either no further weight gain as height increases, or weight gain that is slower than height gain. However, children over 7 years old with obesity and/or complications may benefit from gradual weight loss of, for example, 0.5 kg per month. Adolescents who have stopped growing and assumed adult proportions should be treated accordingly, in which case weight loss of around 0.5 kg per week may be appropriate.

Appropriate dietary suggestions vary from one child to the next, but might include:

- a balanced, varied diet for the whole family
- meals at regular times; avoid 'grazing' and eating while watching television
- smaller portions (children should not be given adult-sized portions)
- avoid using food/snacks as rewards or treats
- healthy snacks (e.g. fruit) as alternatives to sweets, chocolates, crisps, nuts, biscuits, cakes etc.
- less energy-dense food: semi-skimmed milks, low-fat spreads
- whole foods that take time to eat (e.g. fruits and wholemeal bread)
- at least five portions of fruit and vegetables per day
- low-calorie drinks (preferably water)
- grill, boil or bake foods without added fat, rather than frying.

The UK National Institute of Health and Clinical Excellence (NICE) is recognized internationally as a leader in formulating guidelines for the prevention and management of ill health. The recommendations relating to diet in the recent NICE guidelines for childhood obesity with regard to lifestyle changes are shown in Table 10.1.

Physical activity. Increasing sustainable physical activity is crucial in the management of childhood obesity. The recent NICE guidelines for childhood obesity recommend that children and adolescents spend at least 60 minutes a day on moderate-intensity physical activity (although this may not be enough to prevent obesity), and should take part in activities that improve bone health, muscle strength and flexibility at least twice a week. NICE points out, however, that the amount of activity that children and young people need to prevent obesity is unclear. The RCPCH/NOF guidelines emphasize tailoring activity to the individual child and family.

TABLE 10.1

Recommendations relating to diet included in the recent guidelines for lifestyle changes for childhood obesity developed by the UK National Institute of Health and Clinical Excellence

Nutrient/food	Recommendation
Total fat	Reduce to no more than 35% food energy
Saturated fat	Reduce to no more than 11% food energy
Total carbohydrate	Increase to more than 50% food energy
Sugars (added)	Reduce to no more than 11% food energy
Dietary fiber	Increase non-starch polysaccharides to 18 g per day
Salt	Reduce to no more than 6 g salt per day*
Fruit and vegetables	Increase to at least five portions of a variety of fruit and vegetables per day

*The maximum amount of salt recommended for children is less than that for adults.
These recommendations do not apply to children younger than 2 years of age. Between 2 and 5 years, a flexible approach to the timing and extent of dietary change should be taken. By the age of 5 years, children's diets should be consistent with the recommendations for adults.

- Any increase in activity will help.
- Aim for sustainable lifestyle activity such as walking, cycling, using the stairs instead of lifts.
- Develop an active lifestyle in the whole family.
- Walk or cycle to school.
- Encourage active play that is enjoyable and activities that do not cause embarrassment.
- Decrease TV viewing and other sedentary behaviors.

Secondary care may provide further expertise, and more structured and intensive management of overweight/obese children. Residential weight-loss camps ('fat camps') can be successful means of inducing weight loss but will only produce long-term benefits if sustainable behavioral techniques are a fundamental element of the program (e.g. Carnegie camps for children in the UK provide young people and their families with multidisciplinary re-education and support, including cognitive behavior therapy). Behavioral therapy is integral in programs such as MEND and the Carnegie initiative in order to sustain long-term benefits.

Pharmacotherapy. Orlistat or sibutramine can be prescribed for children aged 12 years and older with physical or severe psychological comorbidities. However, this must be done in a specialist pediatric setting by a multidisciplinary team with experience in this age group who can provide expertise in drug monitoring, psychological support, behavioral interventions and physical activity. Once established, drug treatment can be continued in primary care settings, depending on local circumstances and licensing or guidelines.

Bariatric surgery. Adolescents may be considered for bariatric surgery in rare and extreme circumstances, but must have achieved physiological maturity. They will normally have attempted and failed with standard first-line weight-loss techniques. Surgery is normally done in adult surgical units with specialist pediatric support.

Severely obese children and their families who are considering surgery should discuss the potential benefits and longer-term implications of surgery, as well as the associated risks, in detail with the primary care team who will be involved in their long-term care as well as with the clinicians responsible for their in-patient treatment.

Comprehensive psychological, education, family and social assessment beforehand is a prerequisite. The psychological implications of bariatric surgery are discussed on pages 117–18.

Preventative initiatives. As healthcare professionals deal with the clinical manifestations of the obesity epidemic one patient at a time, it would be reassuring to know that drivers for environmental change are occurring simultaneously. In the UK there are important initiatives or proposals for change, such as:

- no advertising of or sponsorship by inappropriate products in television programs aimed at preschool children (< 5 years old)
- a range of rules aimed at the content of all food and drink advertising, designed to reduce its impact on children generally, and to avoid targeting certain techniques at some age groups altogether.

A Cochrane review of childhood anti-obesity initiatives was unenthusiastic about their benefits, concluding that although many diet and exercise interventions aimed at preventing childhood obesity promote healthy diets and increase physical activity, they do not appear to have radical impacts on reducing overweight and obesity. It also highlighted the lack of quality data on the effects of programs to tackle childhood obesity.

Clearly, better initiatives are needed if the rising tide of childhood obesity is to be reversed.

The elderly

With increasing age, there is a redistribution of body fat to the abdomen and loss of muscle mass (sarcopenia).

Assessment. Because of the decrease in skeletal muscle mass and the redistribution of body fat, the use of BMI to assess obesity in the elderly may be misleading. Waist circumference is a more useful measure since intra-abdominal fat is clearly related to increased morbidity and mortality. Determination of sarcopenic obesity requires precise methods of measuring fat and lean components simultaneously, such as dual-energy X-ray absorptiometry. For clinical purposes, the measurement of waist:hip ratio (WHR) may serve this purpose (see pages 19–20), and relates particularly well to cardiometabolic risk.

Consequences. Although a high BMI may be associated with decreased mobility in the elderly, it has a smaller effect on overall and cardiovascular mortality. The risks of obesity in old age increase when the fat is predominantly visceral and when sarcopenia is also present; and this group of individuals are most affected by frailty and disability with increasing age. Overall mortality is more likely to increase when the BMI decreases. Prior weight history may also be an important predictor of risk; older, heavier people who gained more than 10% of midlife bodyweight or thinner, older people who had lost 10% or more of bodyweight have a higher risk than thinner people with stable weight. Being overweight or obese in young adulthood and underweight or obese in later life increases the risk of premature death in old age.

Compared with normal-weight people, both underweight and obese older adults report impaired quality of life, and poorer physical functioning and physical well-being. Obesity-related diseases (diabetes, hypertension, dementia) are increasing in the elderly, as in younger individuals.

Obesity-related disability. There is a positive association between fat mass and disability. Fat mass also predicts disability 3 years later, independent of low fat-free mass, age, physical activity or chronic disease. A high BMI is a strong predictor of long-term risk for mobility disability in older women, a risk that persists to very old age. Increased waist circumference is also a predictor for most disability outcomes, and sarcopenic obesity at baseline is particularly predictive of disability in activities of daily living at 8 years' follow-up. Obesity is a significant independent predictor for older persons being housebound, and losing independence, particularly when associated with an unhealthy diet and physical inactivity. A paradoxic increase in risk of disability has been associated with weight loss in very elderly women (whether from normal or overweight); both obesity and underweight are strongly associated with the development of frailty.

Impaired glucose tolerance and type 2 diabetes. The prevalence of type 2 diabetes increases progressively with age. Increased body fatness and abdominal obesity, rather than aging per se, are thought to be directly linked to the greatly increased incidence of type 2 diabetes among the elderly. Nevertheless, there is evidence that insulin secretion decreases with age even after adjustments for differences in adiposity, fat distribution and physical activity.

Hypertension and cardiovascular disease. Both high blood pressure and cardiovascular risk continue to be highly correlated with obesity, particularly abdominal obesity, even in old age. Irrespective of the presence of other cardiovascular risk factors, those who are obese in middle age have a higher risk of hospitalization and mortality from coronary heart disease, cardiovascular disease and diabetes in older age than those who are normal weight.

Cognitive function. Obesity defined by BMI or waist circumference is associated with poorer cognition in the elderly. Obesity at midlife is associated with an increased risk of dementia and Alzheimer's disease later in life, and clustering of vascular risk factors increases the risk in an additive manner.

A larger WHR may be related to neurodegenerative, vascular or metabolic processes that affect brain structures, underlying cognitive decline and dementia.

Management. For overweight elderly individuals in good health, there is no good evidence to show that weight loss reduces mortality risk. Specific weight-loss recommendations may be unnecessary even among overweight persons with one or more obesity-related health conditions (e.g. hypertension, dyslipidemia, insulin resistance, glucose intolerance), which can be ameliorated independently of weight loss.

In the overweight (but not obese) elderly, weight fluctuation, in any direction and irrespective of intention, may increase the risk for mobility limitation. It is desirable to prevent weight gain, particularly among the obese, and weight loss, particularly among the non-obese.

While the benefits of weight loss in the elderly are uncertain, it has been shown that self-selected obese older women can achieve a moderate weight loss and increase in physical activity that results in short-term improvements in physical performance, self-reported function, vitality, and life quality outcomes. The North American

Society of the Study of Obesity has taken the position that weight loss improves physical function and quality of life, and reduces the medical complications associated with obesity in older persons.

Diet. In general it is not appropriate to advise caloric restriction as the primary modality to induce weight loss, although it may be appropriate where mobility is the major problem. The overall diet must be balanced and contain adequate protein. It is generally appropriate to advise a reduction in intake of saturated fat, to increase fiber and to ensure that the diet contains sufficient micronutrients. There are clear benefits in optimizing the intake of vitamin D and calcium in the elderly. Omega-3 fatty acids reduce the risk of cardiovascular events, and may have benefits for the maintenance of cognitive function; several clinical trials are under way and preliminary data are promising.

Physical activity. Increased physical activity is preferable to diet-induced weight loss, other than in those with predominantly obesity-related mobility disorders, and also has beneficial effects on muscle strength, endurance and overall well-being. Exercise regimens that include strength training have benefits over and above those focusing on endurance training alone; such programs are feasible and safe.

Pharmacotherapy and bariatric surgery. Little is known about the benefits of drugs for inducing weight loss in the elderly, since most clinical trials exclude older patients. Bariatric surgery, and Roux-en-Y gastric bypass (see page 107) in particular, can be safely performed in selected patients over 70 years of age, and has the same benefits as for younger subjects. Although morbidity and mortality are increased in the elderly, the risk:benefit ratio is considered acceptable, particularly in those who have severe obesity-related comorbidities and restricted mobility.

It is most important that an active lifestyle is promoted from an early age and maintained through adulthood to prevent substantial weight gain and obesity with age.

Pregnant women

In Australia, approximately 35% of women aged between 25 and 35 years are overweight or obese.

Risks. The major risks of obesity to the pregnant woman and newborn are shown in Table 10.2. As shown, these all increase with increasing BMI. While there is an extensive body of literature related to defining the problems and potential complications associated with obesity during pregnancy and childbirth, information relating to effective interventions that may be implemented to improve maternal, fetal and infant health outcomes is lacking.

Management. Obese women who gained less than 8 kg during pregnancy had lower rates of large-for-gestational age babies, pre-eclampsia, cesarean section and operative vaginal birth. However, women with high weight gain during pregnancy had an increased rate of cesarean section in each of the five BMI categories.

Restriction of weight gain in pregnancy increases the incidence of preterm birth in women with a normal BMI, but not in women with a BMI above 26 kg/m^2. Based on current evidence, it is generally recommended that overweight and obese women avoid weight loss during pregnancy but weight gain should be limited to approximately 5 kg. Overweight and obese women treated with dietary and exercise advice have a significant reduction in macrosomia without any increase in small-for-gestational age infants.

Nutrition. Women who consume a 'cafeteria style' diet with a high glycemic index (GI; see page 73) have babies with more body fat than women who consume a low-GI diet during pregnancy. A low-GI diet was associated with lower maternal HbA_{1c} in pregnancy, and with lower birth weight, the benefit persisting to at least 5 years of age. A reduction in caloric intake is not unreasonable provided the diet is healthy and balanced and ketosis avoided.

Physical activity. Household and care-giving activity constitute 24–40% of total energy expenditure in each trimester. Median total energy expenditure decreases in the third trimester compared with the first and second trimesters. Vigorous leisure activity during the first two

TABLE 10.2

Risk of health outcomes by maternal body mass index (BMI) groupings

Health outcome	Maternal BMI		
	25.01–30.00	30.01–40.00	> 40.01
Mother			
Hypertension	1.74 (1.45–2.15)	3.00 (2.40–3.74)	4.87 (3.27–7.24)
Gestational diabetes	1.78 (1.25–2.52)	2.95 (2.05–4.25)	7.44 (4.42–12.54)
Cesarean section	1.50 (1.36–1.66)	2.02 (1.79–2.28)	2.54 (1.94–3.32)
Baby			
Stillbirth	1.16 (0.62–2.17)	1.19 (0.56–2.55)	0.89 (0.12–6.60)
Birth defect	1.26 (0.85–1.87)	1.58 (1.02–2.46)	3.41 (1.67–6.94)
Neonatal hypoglycemia	0.78 (0.36–1.66)	2.57 (1.39–4.78)	7.14 (3.04–16.74)
Neonatal jaundice	1.02 (0.92–1.12)	0.98 (0.88–1.13)	1.44 (1.09–1.89)
Preterm birth (< 34 weeks)	1.22 (0.90–1.64)	1.16 (0.81–1.67)	2.13 (1.13–4.01)
Admission to NICU	0.92 (0.73–1.16)	1.25 (0.97–1.62)	2.77 (1.81–4.25)

Values are odds ratios (with 95% confidence intervals in parentheses). NICU, neonatal intensive care unit. Data from Callaway et al. 2006.

trimesters has been associated with a reduction in preterm birth and favorably affects the outcome of labor. Benefits for the offspring include reduced fat mass at birth and in childhood. The benefit of introducing exercise during pregnancy for previously sedentary women remains to be established, however.

Key points – specific patient groups

- Management of obesity is different for different age groups.
- There are specific benefits but also specific risks if treatment is inappropriate.
- In childhood obesity the aim is usually to attenuate weight gain rather than induce weight loss.
- An elderly person at any given body mass index or waist circumference is always likely to have a higher percentage of fat.

Key references

Callaway LK, Prins JB, Chang AM, McIntyre HD. The prevalence and impact of overweight and obesity in an Australian obstetric population. *Med J Aust* 2006;184:56–9.

Dean H, Flett B. Natural history of type 2 diabetes diagnosed in childhood; long term follow-up in young adult years. *Diabetes* 2002;51(suppl 1):A24(Abstract).

Dietz WH. Health consequences of obesity in youth: childhood predictors of adult disease. *Pediatrics* 1998;101(3 Pt 2):518–25.

Gibson P, Edmunds L, Haslam DW, Poskitt E. *An Approach to Weight Management in Children and Adolescents (2–18 years) in Primary Care.* Royal College of Paediatrics and Child Health and National Obesity Forum. http://nationalobesityforum.org.uk/images/stories/W_M_guidelines/Children_and_adolescents.pdf

Leeds Carnegie. *Try rugby – tackling social issues in Yorkshire.* www.leedscarnegie.co.uk/news_C4EC090C6B2E426298502D6C17547F57.htm

MEND. *Programmes to help children become fitter, healthier and happier.* www.mendprogramme.org

NICE. *Obesity: Guidance on the Prevention, Identification, Assessment and Management of Overweight and Obesity in Adults and Children.* CG43. London: National Institute for Health and Clinical Excellence, 2006. www.nice.org.uk/nicemedia/pdf/CG43NICEGuideline.pdf

Oude Luttikhuis H, Baur L, Jansen H et al. Interventions for treating obesity in children. *Cochrane Database Syst Rev* 2009;issue 1: CD001872. www.thecochranelibrary.com

Roubenoff R. Sarcopenia and its implications for the elderly. *Eur J Clin Nutr* 2000;54(suppl 3):S40–7.

A plethora of online tools, publications and weight-loss programs are available for the management of obesity at both an individual level in clinical practice and on a larger scale within the community. A selection of these management tools are discussed below.

OBEMAN

Managing obesity in clinical practice is often complex and time consuming. Obeman (www.obeman.com) is a commercial step-by-step computer program, designed by one of the authors (G. Wittert), to help healthcare professionals with the management of obese and overweight patients. Obeman provides:

- information on treatment options, including lifestyle change, meal replacements, low-calorie diets, medication and surgery
- tools tailored to health professionals (evidence-based information, links to peer-reviewed articles, practical management tips) and patients (fact sheets, food and activity diaries, healthy eating guides)
- practical and effective lifestyle programs, including nutrition, activity, behavior management and counseling.

Following the initial consultation, the patient's history, management plan and progress to date can be reviewed at each visit, and weight and waist circumference updated. Additional support for a particular management approach is then provided or a new action can be chosen. A menu of actions is provided, each of which takes 5–10 minutes to implement; a built-in 'expert' asks questions and provides information and advice about how to proceed. At the end of the consultation the program provides a prompt to schedule the next appointment with the patient to review the outcome and implement the next step.

Rather than using a linear approach, the Obeman program allows management to start at any point (diet, physical activity, education, etc.) depending on the requirements of the patient. It also enables construction of an appropriate care plan and can be used to generate referral letters and personalized dietary and exercise advice.

EPODE

EPODE is an obesity prevention program that aims to integrate healthier lifestyles into daily life. The aim is engagement of all relevant local stakeholders in a coordinated whole-community approach to promote healthy behaviors, and to minimize unhealthy behaviors, through environmental change, supported by a positive, concrete and stepwise learning process. The integration of nutritional education into the school curriculum, for example, can change the dietary behavior of children and their families. By creating changes in group dynamics, changes in social norms occur, leading to healthier lifestyles. Since its inception in France in 2003 the program has expanded throughout France and is now active in Spain and Belgium and is also being implemented elsewhere in Europe, Canada and Australia.

The involvement of, and part funding by, industry stakeholders has been somewhat controversial, but in reality this has not been problematic and a strict ethical charter is adhered to. Since the start of the EPODE campaign to 2007, the prevalence of overweight and obesity has declined substantially across the towns involved.

Counterweight

Counterweight is an evidence-based weight management program for use in primary care. It is currently provided throughout Scotland and in an increasing number of UK primary care trusts.

The model is based on weight management advisers: dietitians specializing in obesity management who train and support primary practice staff to incorporate the program into existing healthcare services. Locally employed 'buddy' dietitians take over responsibility once the model has been implemented.

The objective of the Counterweight program is to achieve and maintain a medically valuable weight loss of 5–10% for as many people as possible, starting with lifestyle intervention. Patients can choose between a goal-setting approach, a structured prescribed eating plan or a group program, all based on 500–600 kcal daily energy deficit. Patients also receive advice on increasing physical activity, and behavioral strategies are a core component of the model. The program is flexible and can be delivered individually or to families or groups, depending on need and available resources. Each patient is recommended to have nine appointments of 10–30 minutes in the first year.

Second-line interventions may include the use of anti-obesity medications and referral to a dietitian, psychologist or secondary care services. Weight maintenance is encouraged either following weight loss or as the first option with particular groups of patients.

Although developed for implementation in primary care trusts, Counterweight can be adapted for use in other settings – in Scotland there is some interest in providing the service through community pharmacy.

Evaluation. Mean weight reductions at 12 months were 3.0 kg in all patients (n = 684) and 4.3 kg in high attenders (n = 422), and at 24 months were 2.4 kg in all patients (n = 391) and 3.3 kg in high attenders (n = 225). Overall, 30% of all patients enrolled and followed up in the program, and almost 40% of high attenders maintained weight loss of at least 5% at 12 months.

MEND

MEND is a childhood obesity management program developed by the UK Institute of Child Health and Great Ormond Street Hospital. MEND is a community, family-based multidisciplinary program for overweight and obese children aged between 7 and 12 years and their families. It places equal emphasis on (M)ind, (E)xercise, (N)utrition and (D)iet (although the 'D' now stands for 'do it!'). It combines all the elements known to be vital in treating and preventing overweight or obesity in children, including family involvement, practical education in nutrition and diet, increasing physical activity and behavioral change. The program comprises 18 2-hour sessions over 9 weeks, featuring mind, nutrition or diet learning and an hour of enjoyable land- or water-based exercise. Theory sessions emphasize practical hands-on learning using specially designed games, visual demonstrations and activities, including a supermarket tour and recipe tasting. The program is backed by the evidence of a randomized control trial, and is reproducible in any area by virtue of its carefully and accurately annotated protocol.

Care pathways

Figure 11.1 shows the care pathway developed by the UK National Obesity Forum (NOF). The pathway emphasizes that although more complex modalities are used as levels of obesity increase, treatments are still implemented alongside lifestyle methods.

The NOF model for the management of obesity is based on that of the Rotherham Institute for Obesity (RIO). Rotherham is an obesity hot spot in the North of England, with a high level of deprivation and amongst the worst levels of excess weight and comorbidities in the UK. The institute uses a fully integrated traditional four-tier model for obesity management (Figure 11.2), within which individuals can move between tiers as appropriate. Preoperative care of bariatric patients is also undertaken within the institute. It recently beat 4000 candidates for the NHS award for excellence in commissioned services.

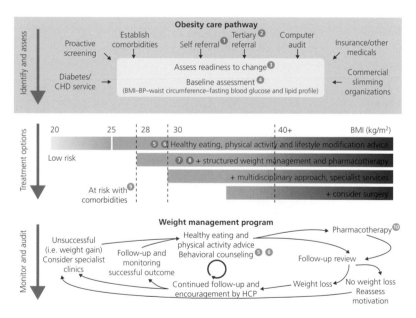

Figure 11.1 Obesity care pathway developed by the UK National Obesity Forum. BMI, body mass index; BP, blood pressure; CHD, coronary heart disease; HCP, healthcare professional.

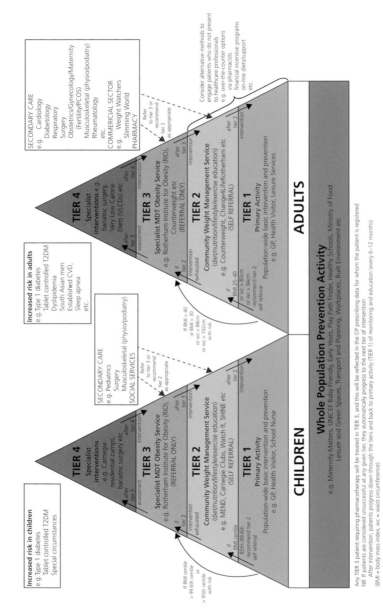

Figure 11.2 The NOF four-tier model for management of obesity in children and adults, integrating obesity management within the community and within the surgery environment (by the multidisciplinary team), with specialist medical obesity management and bariatric surgery.

Key points – management tools and programs

- There are successful models for every stage of obesity, including prevention, childhood obesity and the treatment and management of adult obesity.
- The National Obesity Forum model, which has won the prestigious NHS award for commissioned services, can potentially be implemented anywhere.
- There is robust evidence indicating the effectiveness of the MEND program for children and the Counterweight program for adults.

Key references

EPODE (Belgium). www.viasano.be

EPODE (France). www.epode.fr

EPODE (Spain). www.thaoweb.com

Laws R; Counterweight Project Team. A new evidence-based model for weight management in primary care: the Counterweight Programme. *J Hum Nutr Diet* 2004;17:191–208. *also see* www.counterweight.org

OBEMAN Obesity Management System. www.obeman.com

Sacher PM, Chadwick P, Kolotourou M et al. The MEND study: sustained improvements on health outcomes in obese children at one year. *Obesity* 2007;15:A92. www.mendprogramme .org/sites/default/files/MEND/RCT_ Data_071021.pdf *also see* www.mendprogramme.org

Useful resources

UK
British Obesity and Metabolic
Surgery Society
info@british-obesity-surgery.org
www.british-obesity-surgery.org

British Obesity Surgery Patient
Association
Tel: 08456 02 04 46
enquiries@BOSPA.org
www.bospa.org

Diabetes UK
Tel: +44 (0)20 7424 1000
info@diabetes.org.uk
www.diabetes.org.uk

National Obesity Forum
Tel: +44 (0)115 846 2109
info@nof.uk.com
www.nationalobesityforum.org.uk

Royal College of Paediatrics and
Child Health
Tel: +44 (0)20 7092 6000
www.rcph.ac.uk

USA
American Diabetes Association
AskADA@diabetes.org
www.diabetes.org

American Society for Metabolic
and Bariatric Surgery
Tel: +1 352 331 4900
info@asmbs.org
www.asmbs.org

The Obesity Society (USA)
Tel: +1 301 563 6526
www.obesity.org

International
Australian and New Zealand
Obesity Society
office@asso.org.au
http://asso.org.au

European Association for the
Study of Diabetes
Tel: +49 211 758 4690
secretariat@easd.org
www.easd.org

International Association for the
Study of Obesity
(includes the International Obesity
Taskforce)
Tel: +44 (0)20 7467 9610
obesity@iotf.org
www.iotf.org
www.iaso.org

Index